Praise for *The Body Ecology Diet*

"Body Ecology emphasizes the importance of what we put into our bodies and teaches a way of eating that makes me feel like I am in control of my health and in tune with my body's intuitive needs. Cultured vegetables and coconut kefir have become essentials, not only in my home, but whenever I travel."

— **Jessica Biel,** actress

—∿∿—

"No one has ever put together all that we need to know about recovering and enhancing immunity—until now. I am making it 'must reading' for all my patients with candidiasis, immune disorders, and food allergies."

— **Keith W. Sehnert, M.D.,** author of *Selfcare/Wellcare* and *Stress/Unstress* and coauthor of *Beyond Antibiotics*

—∿∿—

*"Donna Gates puts kefir and other naturally cultured foods back on the map in **The Body Ecology Diet**. Must reading for anyone battling candida and other digestive problems."*

— **Sally Fallon,** author of *Nourishing Traditions* and President of the Weston A. Price Foundation

—∿∿—

*"**The Body Ecology Diet** takes the mystery out of the often-confusing topic of eating for optimum health. Donna Gates's book combines recent scientific thought with proven traditional healing concepts and common sense . . ."*

— **Michael A. Schmidt, N.D.** author of *Tired of Being Tired* ... *biotics*

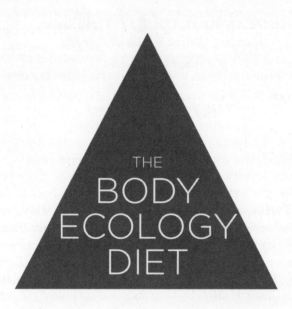

THE
BODY
ECOLOGY
DIET

Hay House Titles of Related Interest

―⁓―

YOU CAN HEAL YOUR LIFE, the movie,
starring Louise L. Hay & Friends
(available as a 1-DVD program and an expanded 2-DVD set)
Watch the trailer at: **www.LouiseHayMovie.com**

THE SHIFT, the movie,
starring Dr. Wayne W. Dyer
(available as a 1-DVD program and an expanded 2-DVD set)
Watch the trailer at: **www.DyerMovie.com**

―⁓―

*ARE YOU TIRED AND WIRED?: Your Proven 30-Day Program
for Overcoming Adrenal Fatigue and Feeling Fantastic,*
by Marcelle Pick, MSN, OB/GYN NP

*THE BODY "KNOWS": How to Tune In to Your Body and Improve
Your Health,* by Caroline Sutherland

*AWAKENING TO THE SECRET CODE OF YOUR MIND:
Your Mind's Journey to Inner Peace,* by Dr. Darren R. Weissman

*JUST AN OUNCE OF PREVENTION . . . Is Worth a Pound of
Cure: A Modern Guide to Healthful Living from the Originator of
the Blood-Type Diet,* by Dr. James L. D'Adamo, with
Allan Richards

*THE PERFECT GENE DIET: Use Your Body's Own Apo E
Gene to Treat High Cholesterol, Weight Problems, Heart Disease,
Alzheimer's . . . and More!* by Pamela McDonald, NP

*RAW BASICS: Incorporating Raw Living Foods into Your Diet
Using Easy and Delicious Recipes,* by Jenny Ross

―⁓―

All of the above are available at your local bookstore,
or may be ordered by visiting:

Hay House UK: **www.hayhouse.co.uk**
Hay House USA: **www.hayhouse.com**®
Hay House Australia: **www.hayhouse.com.au**
Hay House South Africa: **www.hayhouse.co.za**
Hay House India: **www.hayhouse.co.in**

THE
BODY
ECOLOGY
DIET

Recovering Your Health and
Rebuilding Your Immunity

DONNA GATES
WITH LINDA SCHATZ

HAY HOUSE

Australia • Canada • Hong Kong • India
South Africa • United Kingdom • United States

First published and distributed in the United Kingdom by:
Hay House UK Ltd, 292B Kensal Rd, London W10 5BE. Tel.: (44) 20 8962 1230;
Fax: (44) 20 8962 1239. www.hayhouse.co.uk

Published and distributed in the United States of America by:
Hay House, Inc., PO Box 5100, Carlsbad, CA 92018-5100. Tel.: (1) 760 431 7695
or (800) 654 5126; Fax: (1) 760 431 6948 or (800) 650 5115. www.hayhouse.com

Published and distributed in Australia by:
Hay House Australia Ltd, 18/36 Ralph St, Alexandria NSW 2015.
Tel.: (61) 2 9669 4299; Fax: (61) 2 9669 4144. www.hayhouse.com.au

Published and distributed in the Republic of South Africa by:
Hay House SA (Pty), Ltd, PO Box 990, Witkoppen 2068.
Tel./Fax: (27) 11 467 8904. www.hayhouse.co.za

Published and distributed in India by:
Hay House Publishers India, Muskaan Complex, Plot No.3, B-2, Vasant Kunj,
New Delhi – 110 070. Tel.: (91) 11 4176 1620; Fax: (91) 11 4176 1630.
www.hayhouse.co.in

Distributed in Canada by:
Raincoast, 9050 Shaughnessy St, Vancouver, BC V6P 6E5. Tel.: (1) 604 323 7100;
Fax: (1) 604 323 2600

A catalogue record for this book is available from the British Library.

ISBN 978-1-8485-0709-8

Printed and bound in Great Britain by TJ International Ltd, Padstow, Cornwall

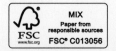

Contents

—⁓—

Appendix A

Appendix B

Figures

1. Dr. Crook's Candida Questionnaire and Score Sheet
2. Expansion/Contraction Continuum
3. Acid/Alkaline Foods
4. Ups and Downs of Cleansing
5. Food Combining Chart
6. 80/20 Rule #1
7. 80/20 Rule #2
8. The Body Ecology Diet Menu Suggestions
9. Body Ecology Diet Simplified

Please Note!

This book synthesizes information from many sources and points of view, including modern medical science, ancient Chinese medicine, naturopathy, and the authors' personal study, observation, and experience. The conclusions expressed herein are those of the authors.

The Body Ecology Diet is written and published as an information resource and educational guide for both professionals and non-professionals. It should not be used as a substitute for your physician's advice. Be sure to work with a physician who knows the importance of diet in healing and who has experience in treating Candida Related Complex and other immune disorders. While we endorse the Body Ecology Diet and related recommendations, you should make your decision based on all the information at hand, knowing that you are the primary force in directing your own life and health.

Preface

This Book Is For . . .

- People who have symptoms of a weak immune system and want to boost their immunity.

- Holistic health-care practitioners whose clients have candidiasis or other immune-system deficiencies. Your clients will thrive on the Body Ecology Diet and get more out of their sessions with you.

- Doctors who prescribe antibiotics, birth-control pills, radiation, chemotherapy, cortisone, steroids, etc. The Body Ecology Diet will help your patients avoid an overgrowth of harmful yeast during therapy and then help them restore their inner ecosystems and prevent future illness.

You Should Read This Book If . . .

- You suspect or know you have candidiasis (CRC), chronic fatigue syndrome, cancer, AIDS, or other immune-system deficiencies.

- You have known or suspected food allergies or frequent digestive problems.

- You have frequent skin rashes, constipation, or PMS.

- You are bothered by headaches, or muscle or joint pains.

- You always seem to be tired, nervous, or depressed, or your memory seems to be poor.

- You are sensitive to tobacco, perfume, or other chemical odors.

- You have taken birth-control pills.

- You have been plagued and frustrated by symptoms that persist no matter what you do to get rid of them.

- You have a history of drug use, including extensive use of antibiotics or illegal drugs.

- You want to ensure the health of your children and other loved ones.

- You want to prevent major disease that doesn't manifest until years after the seeds have been sown: cancer, AIDS, heart disease.

—∿∿∿—

Candidiasis and Its Relation to AIDS, Cancer, Chronic Fatigue, and Other Immune Disorders

Welcome to the Body Ecology Diet (B.E.D.), a proven way to enhance your health and clear up the symptoms of candidiasis—an overgrowth of yeast. As long as a candida overgrowth exists in your body, the immune system is so overwhelmed that it cannot even begin to do its real job, which is to fight invaders such as HIV, herpes, or rebellious groups of cells (cancer). Candidiasis reflects an immune system under siege; and until you bring the candidiasis under control through diet, rest, exercise, and a determined attitude, other immune-compromised conditions cannot be conquered. We need to focus on the candida as the first step to improving immunity. So while this book is written specifically for people with candidiasis, it is just as valuable for those with related immune-compromised conditions.

The Body Ecology Diet (or "The Diet") offers a framework for the rest of your life. It provides basic tools that will help you restore and maintain the balance and vitality your body deserves. It goes *with* the flow of nature, not against it. It strengthens your immunity. The Diet can bring a greater sense of calm to your life by providing clear guidelines and principles.

Does this mean you'll never eat pizza, hamburgers, or dessert again? Not necessarily! In its strictest, therapeutic form, The Diet is designed to heal a serious, life-threatening inner imbalance. If you have the willpower to follow it for three months to a year (depending on the severity of your imbalance), you will become well . . . well enough to eat those foods again (although not to excess). In grappling with candida to regain your health, you will become sensitive to the needs of your body. You will learn what works and what doesn't, and you will start appreciating the value of healthy eating. You will adapt The Diet to your lifestyle, inventing your own recipes and favorite food combinations. You will even enjoy the special desserts we've created.

At first, The Diet limits the foods you can have, but as your health improves, you can try a wider variety of healthy foods. Then occasional divergence even from these foods will not do the harm it does now. If some of your symptoms reappear, you'll be able to return to the basic Diet and get yourself back on an even keel.

Tips for Reading and Mastering the Body Ecology Diet

There's a lot of information packed into these pages! You'll be excited to find answers to your health concerns—but you'll probably be overwhelmed by all the things to know and do as you begin The Diet. Don't worry—everything will fall into place once you start experimenting with the foods on The Diet.

Read the book all the way through, highlighting the ideas and actions you consider important. Then, once you've *completed* the book and started on The Diet, go back and highlight in a *different* color, because you'll have a different point of view.

You may find that some information is repeated in different chapters and sections. That's because we believe it's important enough to be emphasized in more than one place. Now, allow us to introduce ourselves, and then let's begin. . . .

Donna's Story

"A long path of study, experimentation, prayer, and faith has brought me to the point where I am today: a healthy, optimistic woman who wants to share what I've learned. But to reach this point, I've been through many ups and downs in my campaign to overcome candidiasis, a condition that saps the very core of one's vitality and well-being.

"I was born with a sensitive constitution, including an allergy to milk. I had constant lung problems and colds. When my skin broke out during my teen years, I started taking antibiotics. My skin was very yellow, I had low energy, and sometimes I'd be very 'spacey' for no apparent reason. The antibiotics led to food allergies and digestive problems—and my skin didn't clear up unless I took the antibiotics every day. I went to a dermatologist and complained that the antibiotics made my stomach burn and gave me indigestion, but he said not to worry: people stay on antibiotics for years without problems.

"I was vain, so I did stick with the antibiotics until I was in my 30s. Yet I knew something was wrong, and with my very sensitive body, I had clues it was connected to the food I was eating. So I began my intensive search for answers.

"I tried macrobiotics, natural hygiene, raw foods, and megavitamin therapy. I studied with some of the greatest teachers in these disciplines. Everything I did improved my health somewhat, but not completely. Finally, deeply frustrated, I 'let go' and prayed for help. It was then that I met Dr. William Crook.

"Dr. Crook was a pioneer in treating people with candidiasis, and his books have helped millions. I learned from him, as I had from all my other teachers to date, but still even he did not have the final answers. So, after six years of relentless searching, using the most important truths from all I studied, I developed the Body Ecology Diet, which goes beyond all these disciplines to really set you up forever with a balanced, inner ecology, and I founded a nutrition company called Body Ecology, Inc.

I've learned how we strayed from the optimal health that our Creator intended for us, and how we can return there.

"Everyone who has faithfully followed the Body Ecology Diet has improved dramatically, and I am thrilled to share it with you. I'm confident this book will change your life. If your immune system has weakened to the point where you've developed candidiasis, and you've spent a lot of money, time, and effort to find a cure, I promise you that the Body Ecology Diet will be the end of your search."

Donna Gates
Atlanta, Georgia

Linda's Story

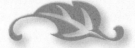

"The Body Ecology Diet has helped lift me out of the worst nightmare of my life. When I met Donna, I had spent nearly four years trying to figure out why I was plagued with persistent symptoms of vaginitis, headaches, food allergies, and urinary and G.I. upsets. I had been to many doctors, tried traditional and non-traditional medicines and regimens, spent hundreds and hundreds of dollars—and I still wasn't symptom free. I had eliminated all sugar, alcohol, and dairy from my diet; taken umpteen vitamin and mineral supplements; and tried internal cleansing cures until I was blue in the face. I was exercising regularly and had learned relaxation techniques.

"I was probably the healthiest sick person around. But until I started The Diet, my symptoms continued. Then I learned from Donna how to use the principle of food combining and, for me, this was the key to accelerating the rate of my improvement.

"I was so tired of doing things that didn't work, that when I found something that did, I went at it with a vengeance. I tried to do absolutely everything Donna teaches. She says to make vegetable soup—I ate it even though mine consistently turned out mediocre. She advocates having soup for breakfast—I did it.

"I'm thrilled to report that most of my symptoms have disappeared, and the rest are under control. At this writing, my health remains excellent, I'm reintroducing, different foods into my diet, and, for the first time in several years, I'm at peace with my body.

"The Diet's recipes *really* helped. At first, it was difficult to change my way of thinking about menus and meals, but after a short while it became second nature. This book represents Donna's many years of accumulated knowledge and application; everything she says is valuable and pertinent. She and I are committed to making improvements in your health, so we ask you to read this book carefully and follow the suggestions and guidelines. Here's to your health!"

Linda Schatz
Alexandria, Virginia

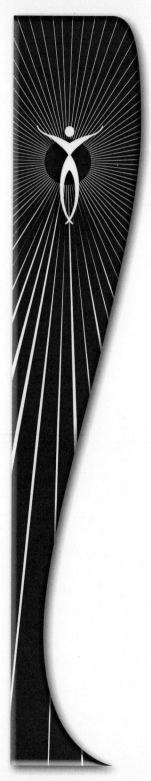

PART I

Introduction:
A Silent Spring
Within

Chapter 1

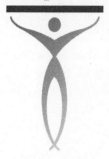

Outer Ecology, Inner Ecology

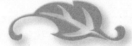

Many years ago, Rachel Carson, author of *Silent Spring*, warned that we are slowly destroying the ecological balance of our planet by adding chemicals to our crops. She spoke out against the pesticides that seep into our food and water supplies, affecting our health and the health of future generations.

In a similar manner, we are destroying the delicate balance of the ecosystem that exists within our own bodies. This intricate ecosystem is inhabited by microorganisms that play an important role in keeping us looking young and feeling healthy and strong. These friendly creatures, known as lactic bacteria, reside in the digestive tract, strengthen the immune system, and help the body defend against "unfriendly" bacteria and the pathogens that cause disease.

In fact, both friendly and unfriendly microorganisms are always present in our bodies, but when we are healthy, the friendly greatly outnumber the unfriendly, keeping our inner ecosystem in harmony. However, many factors weaken our immunity and upset this balance: the chemicals we add to our food and environment, fast-food diets, the stress in our daily lives, and the widespread use of medicines, especially antibiotics and hormones. And when the body is in this weakened state, the unfriendly bacteria can multiply quickly, producing symptoms such as headaches, nausea, skin rashes, and food allergies, as well as other potentially more serious disorders.

This book is about restoring your inner health, strengthening your immune system, and establishing a pattern of living and eating well that will extend your vitality for years to come. The Body Ecology Diet provides basic tools you can use for the rest of your life, tools to help you achieve a new balance in your life. *Anyone*—ill or not—can benefit from The Diet.

It is time to restore the ecology of our planet and the ecology of our bodies. By rebuilding our health and our immunity, we can restore our inner ecology, and we will have a much better chance to achieve all our goals, including restoring the ecology of our outer world.

The Two Faces of Antibiotics

Some 40 years ago, antibiotics ("against life") became the "magic bullets" in curing disease. They were considered miracle drugs. Doctors prescribed antibiotics for such simple maladies as colds and acne. But antibiotics kill not only disease-causing bacteria; they also kill beneficial bacteria, upset the body's inner ecology, and allow unfriendly organisms to take over.

One of the most common types of unfriendly organisms is *Candida albicans*. It is a pathogenic yeast or fungus normally present on inner and outer body surfaces, and it coexists in small numbers in our digestive tract and in a woman's vagina alongside the friendly microorganisms. It thrives when we eat a high-sugar, acid-forming, low-mineral diet. It is an opportunistic organism, and it rapidly takes advantage of any weakness in our system. So if we're eating improperly, taking antibiotics, or changing our chemistry with birth-control pills, we are providing the candida with a perfect environment in which to grab control. The vagina and intestines are especially susceptible, but the fungus can quickly spread into the bloodstream and begin creating colonies of yeast in and on every organ. It is then called a *systemic infection*. Only two days of antibiotic use precipitates candida overgrowth in a susceptible person.[1] When yeast multiplies, it produces toxic waste products, which circulate in the body, poisoning and weakening the immune and endocrine systems.

Symptoms of Candidiasis

The overgrowth of candida constitutes a condition we call candidiasis or Candida Related Complex (CRC). It has been linked to *many* symptoms, including food allergies, digestive disorders, PMS, skin rashes, chronic constipation, recurring headaches, chronic vaginitis, chemical and environmental sensitivities, poor memory, mental fuzziness, and loss of sex drive. CRC occurs side by side with other diseases such as chronic fatigue, cancer, AIDS, Epstein-Barr virus, bronchitis, pneumonia, and immune-system deficiencies. Experts estimate that one in three Americans (higher in younger generations) have candidiasis, but the majority don't attribute their symptoms to this modern epidemic.

To reverse this overgrowth of candida, we must restore an inner environment that prevents candida from taking over. This requires two major actions: killing off the bad yeast and other opportunistic parasitic organisms by creating mineral-rich slightly alkaline blood, and then recolonizing the friendly bacteria and restoring proper digestion. Both are essential to reestablishing your immune system. It won't do any good to reestablish new colonies of friendly bacteria without improving the environment so they can prosper.

A parallel exists in the outer world. Suppose we wanted to revive populations of an endangered species, such as the whooping crane or California condor. We could breed in captivity some of the few remaining birds, then release them into their former territory. But if the conditions endangering them in the first place were not changed (such as inadequate food or contaminated nesting sites), they would not be able to survive or reproduce.

Hurdles in Restoring Your Body Ecology

When antibiotics were first used, they could kill off almost any strain of infection-causing bacteria. But eventually, these bacteria altered their genetic makeup and started resisting the drugs. Now generations of these resisters have multiplied and become even stronger. They have an astounding ability to adjust to different environments. So the task of eliminating them is formidable, but the key is changing the environment so they cannot survive. The Body Ecology Diet improves your inner habitat so that unfriendly organisms cannot predominate.

A parallel to the overuse of antibiotics exists in our excessive use of pesticides. Insects have become resistant to many pesticides, forcing manufacturers to keep changing their formulae. In addition, the pesticides often kill harmless creatures—other insects, birds, animals, and plants. This is comparable to the destruction of friendly bacteria from antibiotics.

Emphasizing Probiotics

Friendly bacteria (also known as probiotics, "for life"), such as lactobacillus, plantarum, and bifidus, and beneficial yeast (*Saccharomyces kefir* and *Torula kefir*) are essential to a wide range of bodily functions. They help white blood cells fight disease, control putrefactive bacteria in the intestines, provide important nutrients for building the blood, assist digestion, protect the intestinal mucosa, prevent diarrhea and constipation, and contribute to bowel elimination. They also manufacture important B vitamins and are the most abundant source of vitamin B-12.

Health-food stores sell bottles of probiotics, which are usually kept in the refrigerator so they won't lose their potency.

Antibiotics should be taken only when absolutely necessary, and when you must take them, stay strictly on The Diet. Start a course of *probi*otics as soon as the *anti*biotic therapy is completed. We'll tell you more about friendly bacteria throughout the book.

How It All Started

Most of us begin life with a clean bill of health, a perfect body inside and out. Experts disagree on exactly where a baby's friendly bacteria come from, but we do know that mother's milk promotes their growth. As breast feeding continues, the bacteria establish themselves in the baby's digestive tract and in the vagina of the female infant. It takes about three months for an inner ecosystem to settle in, and after this period of time, the infant's amount of lactic (friendly) bacteria closely resembles the mother's.

As the child's inner ecology develops, the beneficial bacteria thrive on natural sugars from breast milk, and then from food, particularly complex carbohydrates. These sugars (along with soluble fiber) are the raw materials on which the good microflora act to produce short-chain fatty acids. The body very efficiently uses the salts, or *esters*, of these acids. Acetate and lactate are absorbed and used as fuel. Proprionate travels to the liver and helps regulate cholesterol metabolism. Butyrate helps regulate energy, cholesterol metabolism, and hormone production. It also helps regulate apoptosis (programmed cell death) to prevent colon polyps and cancer.

How Ecosystems Change

Nature gives us two forces to contend with: the process of change, called *succession*; and the constant attempt to return to stability, or *homeostasis*. These occur in our inner as well as our outer worlds.

For example, imagine that during a summer storm lightning sparks a forest fire. Rain extinguishes the fire, and most living creatures leave the site. Then a natural succession begins. The next year, maybe some grass grows in the clearing, and you might see a few butterflies and insects return. A year later, small animals scamper through the meadow. The next summer, shrubs and tree seedlings push up through the ground. Finally, the site becomes woodland again, with its unique balance of plant and animal life. A change occurred—but, in time, there was a gradual return to stability.

When humans grow into puberty and adulthood, the chemistry of the digestive tract changes as well. Our inner ecosystem goes through succession. In infants, certain strains of friendly bacteria predominate, but as we grow older, other types become more common. Yet, throughout, our bodies always attempt to return to homeostasis, to that inner ecological equilibrium.

The things that destroy ecological balance, such as a bulldozer in the woods, or a long-term course of antibiotics, are the factors that give rise to the invasion of new species, which further alter the environment and establish new ecosystems.

When this happens inside us, it lays the foundation for disease to occur.

Benefits of the Body Ecology Diet

The Diet helps restore your inner environment, which in turn will create the basis for a lifetime of true health.

The Diet will help you:
1. Strengthen your organs, digestive tract, and immune system.

2. Starve the yeast.

3. Cleanse your body of waste discarded by the dying yeast.

4. Balance your internal chemistry.

5. Reestablish and feed your inner ecosystem.

The Diet will also help you just plain feel better, physically and mentally. You may have experienced for a short time—or for years—some or all of the symptoms we've mentioned. The Diet and the principles it is built on offer the answers you've been seeking. Now, let's look at the principles of the Body Ecology Diet.

≈

Notes

[1] De Schepper, 1986.

Chapter 2

Overview of the Key Principles of the Body Ecology Diet

The Body Ecology Diet is a synthesis of seven principles of eating and healing. They are pillars of the holistic health field. Some of them are thousands of years old, such as the Chinese concept of yin and yang (contraction/expansion). Others, such as the theory of food combining, are more recent.

The Diet weaves these principles together like pieces in a puzzle. They can create a framework for healthy eating for the rest of your life. They are clear and complementary. This book shows you how to integrate them into your daily routine. When they are properly implemented, you will see your symptoms disappear and your overall health improve.

Principle #1 . . . Expansion/Contraction

Certain foods, such as salt, meat, and poultry, cause the body to contract. Stress also causes a contraction or tightening. When the body is too tight, it cannot function properly: circulation slows down, and elimination of waste comes to a standstill (constipation).

Other foods, like sugar, alcohol, and coffee, cause the body to expand, open up, and relax. People who eat large amounts of contracting foods, such as salt and salty animal foods, crave *expanding* foods in the body's natural attempt to achieve balance. For example, when we eat salty popcorn at the movies, we often return to the refreshment stand for a sweet drink.

A third group of foods, which is neither too contracting nor too expanding, creates a naturally balanced condition in the body. These foods are the cornerstone of The Diet. You will be delighted to learn they are delicious and readily available.

To regain optimal health and an ideal inner ecology, our goal must be to eat foods that balance and complement one another, so we feel neither too contracted nor expanded. The Body Ecology Diet will show you how to do this.

Principle #2 . . . Acid/Alkaline

Acid rain has polluted our forests, lakes, and streams, endangering a wide range of animals and plants. In the same manner, increased acidity due to poor diet has altered our internal chemistry—our pH balance—destroying the beneficial flora of our inner ecosystem.

Illness occurs when our bodies are too acidic and therefore toxic. Understanding how to rebalance our internal chemistry holds a secret to success in healing; restoring the acid/alkaline (pH) balance is essential. The optimal pH for bodily fluids is slightly alkaline. The Body Ecology Diet recommends foods that help alkalize your system, resulting in the proper pH for bodily functions and for beneficial bacteria to flourish.

Principle #3 . . . Uniqueness

When we look at ways to achieve optimal health, we must remember that we are all different. One size does not fit all. A supplement or food that helps one person may not be right for another. We have individual needs and desires. These may change depending on the season, where we live, what food is available, or the current condition of our bodies.

Moreover, we are inundated with nutritional information, much of it confusing and conflicting. We know we should take better care of ourselves, so we try the latest supplement or fad diet, or go back to a well-known routine. The uniqueness principle demystifies this confusion. It points out the strengths and weaknesses of some of the best-known diets, including high protein, raw foods, macrobiotics, and vegetarian. We'll tell you how to adapt them if you have an immune disorder like candidiasis.

With this principle, you will come to trust that the B.E.D. is really a system of health and healing. It is fluid and flexible, yet it also provides excellent guidelines for caring for your body.

Principle #4 . . . Cleansing

This is nature's way of allowing our bodies to get rid of unwanted toxins and foreign substances. Aging blood cells and tissues constantly break down and are replaced by new cells and tissues. The cellular debris must be carried away, and cleansing is the process that does this. A speck of dust gets in your eye, and you start tearing—it's a way to cleanse out the dust. A virus invades your system and you get a cold or fever— it's your immune system at work to drive out the virus. The Diet encourages you to *welcome* cleansings, because they *always* result in a higher level of health and immunity.

Principle #5 . . . Proper Food Combining

This proven system of eating compatible foods at each meal aids digestion and enhances overall health. When you eat foods that don't combine correctly, the digestive system gets mixed signals about which digestive juices and enzymes to release. Food remains in the digestive tract longer than it should, and it starts fermenting. This produces sugars that feed yeast and parasites, and further weakens the digestive tract and immune system.

The rotting food becomes poison, polluting the ecology of your inner world. It's a gruesome image, but it's accurate. As the stagnant food builds up on the walls of the digestive tract, it forms a landscape that only viruses, cancer cells, and parasites can tolerate, just as rats and other scavengers live off city landfills and industrial-waste sites.

Proper food combining greatly reduces gas, bloating, and excess weight. It is essential for establishing a clean, efficient internal environment. You can learn it by following three basic rules, and we'll give plenty of examples and menus.

Principle #6 . . . The 80/20 Principle

When you have candidiasis or other immune-system diseases, it is essential that the food you eat be properly assimilated and then eliminated. A healthy digestive tract is able to do this. But many people weaken their digestive tracts by overeating or eating poorly combined foods. This puts too heavy a workload on the digestive system. The two 80/20 rules guide you in eating moderately to reduce that load.

RULE NUMBER ONE: Eat until your stomach is 80% full, leaving 20% available for digesting. RULE NUMBER TWO: 80% of the food on your plate should be land and/or ocean[2] vegetables. The remaining 20% can be protein or grains and starchy vegetables.

By following the 80/20 and the food-combining principles, you will never again leave the table feeling over-full or bloated.

Principle #7 . . . Step by Step

Everything in nature, in both our inner and outer lives, occurs in a step-by-step, orderly manner. There is no way to avoid this step-by-step process. Because we have not understood and followed this principle, people are not getting well.

You may have spent a great deal of money, effort, and time to feel better, yet are still frustrated, confused, and very concerned about your health. The first steps to wellness are:

- Create a hearty inner ecosystem in your intestines.
- Create energy by nourishing your adrenals and thyroid.
- Conquer any infections . . . especially dangerous fungal infections.
- Cleanse.

You can choose how quickly you progress through the healing process, but you must build this foundation for wellness just as nature does . . . step by step. By the time you finish reading this book, you'll have a good grasp of how to take your own steps toward better health.

Fermented Foods . . . the Missing Link in All Other Systems of Health

Our most brilliant scientists are seeking to identify foods that enhance wellness, yet Body Ecology already recognizes where to find them and how to prepare them. *The new stars of a truly healthy diet are fermented foods!* We ferment vegetables, coconut water, goat's and cow's milk, and the soft spoon-meat in the young coconut. It will take years for other diets to catch up to Body Ecology, and while others still search for answers, we've already put a complete program together for you. You needn't look anywhere else.

Blood Type . . . a Special Key to Wellness

Canadian naturopathic doctors James D'Adamo and his son Peter developed and tested a theory that specifies what foods we should eat and even what type of exercise we need depending on our blood type. Their concept honors our uniqueness, yet they leave out the B.E.D.'s essential focus on establishing a healthy inner ecosystem. You can combine the best features of the blood type and Body Ecology diets by looking at the guidelines we provide.

❧

Notes

[2] See Chapter 12 for a list of ocean vegetables.

Chapter 3

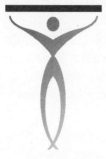

Tips for Success in Using the Body Ecology Diet and This Book

• The B.E.D. is a "how come" as well as a "how to" guide to healthier eating. First, read it through; as you begin grasping the basic principles, this will help your determination to stick to The Diet. Then, begin following it *without becoming overwhelmed* by its many recommendations. The beginning may be difficult for you, because it may be a whole new way of eating and cooking, so do your best, knowing that your reward will be renewed health and vitality. It gets much easier as time goes on. Body Ecology provides you with many wonderful tools to achieve your goal of wellness. You won't be able to pick them all up at one time. You must go step by step.

• Try the recipes we recommend. Most require just a few simple ingredients and not much preparation time. They're nutritious—and delicious!

• This diet works! You could see dramatic results even within the first few days, especially if you have severe symptoms and start attacking them at the point where you'll get the greatest return on your investment of effort. For example, the very first action is to eliminate all forms of sugar from your diet.

• The Diet has helped hundreds of thousands of people overcome conditions that made them feel miserable. Everyone is different, so everyone heals at a different rate. You need to trust the recommendations of The Diet, and—very important— know your body and how it responds.

• Form a support group with others on The Diet. You can trade recipes, solve problems, and hear one another's concerns. This is very valuable, especially in the beginning of your healing.

• Know that eventually you will be able to reintroduce foods not now on The Diet, such as fruits, beans, and additional grains. Be patient.

The Bottom Line:
1. Read the book.
2. Plan menus using foods you like; then shop for these foods.
3. Use the foods in our recipes, always cooking enough for several meals and snacks.
4. Reread the book until the principles are clear.
5. Never give up until you've achieved your goal!

Chapter 4

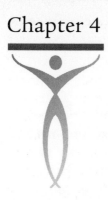

How It All Started

The yeast organism *Candida albicans* has been around for thousands of years, but only in modern times has it overtaken our bodies and compromised our immunity.

Yeast and Fungus: The Silent Invaders

Candida albicans is one of several yeast and fungal organisms present in our bodies. Normally, "friendly bacteria" balance these organisms so they do not grow out of control, and a strong immune system oversees it all. But when we throw our body ecology out of balance due to stress and/or by ingesting sugar, antibiotics, or poor-quality air and water—or compromise our health in other ways—the candida grows out of control and causes a variety of symptoms.

A prominent University of California immunologist, Alan Levin, estimates that one out of three Americans is adversely affected by candida.[3] A single-cell organism, it reproduces asexually and thrives on some of the body's by-products: dead tissue and sugars from food. Unless its source of food is eliminated, it quickly monopolizes entire bodily systems, such as the digestive tract, and can cause mild to severe discomfort. Candida, when it becomes acute, is frequently a major cause of death, especially in victims of cancer and AIDS.

How Do You Know You Have Candidiasis?

From time to time in your life, you've almost certainly had fevers, stomach upsets, ear problems, headaches, skin rashes, aches and pains, and other physical complaints. Normally, these clear up fairly quickly, and the symptoms do not recur frequently. If they do recur, and you go to your doctor with one or several of these complaints but there is no apparent explanation or cure, then you may have a yeast-related condition.

Although researchers are now developing lab tests on blood and feces to diagnose yeast-related conditions, the primary diagnosis methods used to date have been taking a medical history and monitoring response to treatment. Use the questionnaire and score sheet in Figure 1 to help decide if your problems are yeast connected. It was developed by Dr. William Crook, a pioneer in diagnosing and treating candidiasis. The questionnaire is fairly accurate for self-diagnosis of CRC. The best way to figure out whether you have candidiasis is to try the Body Ecology Diet for ten days and observe whether your symptoms begin clearing up.

Candida—A Downward Spiral

Candida overgrowth is a vicious cycle. Our diets are full of sugars that feed the yeast. In women, pregnancy and the use of birth-control pills create hormonal changes that encourage yeast overgrowth. Antibiotics, found extensively in our food supply and prescribed by doctors, kill not only bad bacteria but also the friendly bacteria that normally inhabit our tissues, so this sets up an environment where yeast can multiply uncontrollably. A normal, strong immune system can keep yeast under control. But when yeast do overgrow, they release toxins, which weaken the immune system. At this point, the weakened immune system can no longer defend against germs, so these organisms multiply and quickly invade tissues and organs, causing infections. If you take antibiotics to get rid of these infections, the cycle starts all over.

FIGURE 1

Candida Questionnaire and Score Sheet*

This questionnaire lists factors in your medical history that promote the growth of the common yeast *Candida Albicans* (Section A), and symptoms commonly found in individuals with yeast-connected illness (Sections B and C).

For each yes answer in Section A, circle the Point Score in that section. Total your score, and record it in the box at the end of the section. Then move on to Sections B and C, and score as directed.

Section A: History

	Point Score
1. Have you taken tetracyclines (Sumycin, Panmycin, Vibramycin, Minocin, etc.) or other antibiotics for acne for 1 month (or longer)?	50
2. Have you, at any time in your life, taken other "broad-spectrum" antibiotics for respiratory, urinary, or other infections for 2 months or longer, or for shorter periods 4 or more times in a 1-year span?	50
3. Have you taken a broad-spectrum antibiotic drug – even for one period?	6
4. Have you, at any time in your life, been bothered by persistent prostatitis, vaginitis, or other problems affecting your reproductive organs?	25
5. Have you been pregnant... 2 or more times?	5
1 time?	3
6. Have you taken birth-control pills for...more than 2 years?	15
6 months to 2 years?	8
7. Have you taken prednisone, Decadron, or other cortisone-type drugs by mouth or inhalation** for... more than 2 weeks?	15
2 weeks or less?	6
8. Does exposure to perfumes, insecticides, fabric-shop odors, or other chemicals provoke... moderate to severe symptoms?	20
mild symptoms?	5
9. Are your symptoms worse on damp, muggy days or in moldy places?	20
10. Have you had athlete's foot, ringworm, "jock itch," or other chronic fungal infections of the skin or nails? Have such infections been... severe or persistent?	20
mild or moderate?	10
11. Do you crave sugar?	10
12. Do you crave breads?	10
13. Do you crave alcoholic beverages?	10
14. Does tobacco smoke **really** bother you?	10

Total Score, Section A

*Filling out and scoring this questionnaire should help you and your physician evaluate how *Candida albicans* may be contributing to your health problems. Yet it will not provide an automatic yes or no answer. A comprehensive history and physical examination are important. In addition, laboratory studies, x-rays, and other types of tests may also be appropriate.

**The use of nasal or bronchial sprays containing cortisone and/or other steroids promotes overgrowth in the respiratory tract.

Section B: Major Symptoms

For each symptom that is present, enter the appropriate number in the Point Score column:

    If a symptom is **occasional or mild** ....score **3** points.
    If a symptom is **frequent and/or moderately severe** ....score **6** points.
    If a symptom is **severe and/or disabling** ....score **9** points.

Total the score for this section, and record it in the box at the end of this section.

	Point Score
1. Fatigue or lethargy	
2. Feeling of being "drained"	
3. Poor memory	
4. Feeling "spacey" or "unreal"	
5. Inability to make decisions	
6. Numbness, burning, or tingling	
7. Insomnia	
8. Muscle aches	
9. Muscle weakness or paralysis	
10. Pain and/or swelling in joints	
11. Abdominal pain	
12. Constipation	
13. Diarrhea	
14. Bloating, belching, or intestinal gas	
15. Troublesome vaginal burning, itching, or discharge	
16. Prostatitis	
17. Impotence	
18. Loss of sexual desire or feeling	
19. Endometriosis or infertility	
20. Cramps and/or other menstrual irregularities	
21. Premenstrual tension	
22. Attacks of anxiety or crying	
23. Cold hands or feet and/or chilliness	
24. Shaking or irritability when hungry	
Total Score, Section B	

Section C: Other Symptoms*

For each symptom that is present, enter the appropriate number in the Point Score column:

    If a symptom is **occasional or mild** ....score **3** points.
    If a symptom is **frequent and/or moderately severe** ....score **6** points.
    If a symptom is **severe and/or persistent** ....score **9** points.

Total the score for this section, and record it in the box at the end of this section.

	Point Score
1. Drowsiness	
2. Irritability or jitteriness	
3. Incoordination	
4. Inability to concentrate	
5. Frequent mood swings	
6. Headaches	
7. Dizziness/loss of balance	
8. Pressure above ears…feeling of head swelling	
9. Tendency to bruise easily	
10. Chronic rashes or itching	
11. Psoriasis or recurrent hives	
12. Indigestion or heartburn	
13. Food sensitivity or intolerance	
14. Mucus in stools	
15. Rectal itching	
16. Dry mouth or throat	
17. Rash or blisters in mouth	
18. Bad breath	
19. Foot, hair, or body odor not relieved by washing	
20. Nasal congestion or postnasal drip	

(This section is continued on the next page.)

---

*While the symptoms in this section occur commonly in patients with yeast-connected illness, they also occur commonly in patients who do not have candida.

Section C: Other Symptoms (continued)

For each symptom that is present, enter the appropriate number in the Point Score column:

If a symptom is **occasional or mild** ....score **3** points.
If a symptom is **frequent and/or moderately severe** ....score **6** points.
If a symptom is **severe and/or persistent**..score **9** points.

	Total your score from previous page	
21. Nasal itching		
22. Sore throat		
23. Laryngitis/loss of voice		
24. Cough or recurrent bronchitis		
25. Pain or tightness in chest		
26. Wheezing or shortness of breath		
27. Urinary frequency, urgency, or incontinence		
28. Burning on urination		
29. Spots in front of eyes or erratic vision		
30. Burning or tearing of eyes		
31. Recurrent infections or fluid in ears		
32. Ear pain or deafness		
	Total Score, Section C	
	Total Score, Section B	
	Total Score, Section A	
GRAND TOTAL SCORE (add totals from Sections A, B, and C)		

The Grand Total Score will help you and your physician decide if your health problems are yeast connected. Scores for women will run higher, as 7 items in this questionnaire apply exclusively to women, while only 2 apply exclusively to men.

Yeast-connected health problems are almost certainly present in women with scores **over 180**, and in men with scores **over 140**.

Yeast-connected health problems are probably present in women with scores **over 120**, and in men with scores **over 90**.

Yeast-connected health problems are possibly present in women with scores **over 60**, and in men with scores **over 40**.

With scores less than 60 for women and 40 for men, yeast are less apt to cause health problems.

Questionnaire developed by Dr. William G. Crook, author of *The Yeast Connection* and *Women's Health*, published by Woman's Health Connection (**www.yeastconnection.com**). Used with permission.

Some of the most important current medical research involves the immune system and diseases related to a weak immune response, such as AIDS, Epstein-Barr, cancer, and other serious conditions. Candidiasis is an overgrowth of a serious systemic pathogen. It can be low-grade and chronic or acute and deadly. Its symptoms can mask, overshadow, or accompany other diseases, such as AIDS and cancer. So if your immune system is occupied with dealing with candidiasis, it does not have the strength to fight these other critical illnesses. The good news is that candidiasis can be corrected naturally using the Body Ecology Diet.

Diet Is the Key

Bottom line, getting well is about healthy eating and detoxifying, not taking medicine or vitamin pills. If you don't feed your body with real foods that contain essential proteins, fats, vitamins, and minerals, it will never be strong enough to take over on its own. It will not be able to heal itself as it was created to do. By following the Body Ecology Diet, you will *naturally and easily* regain strength, health, and well-being— and judging from the comments we often receive, you may be surprised to find that you come to really enjoy the delicious foods on The Diet.

A few people still regard candidiasis as a "fad" or fake disease, but this misunderstanding is starting to clear up. Patients whose recurring symptoms and complaints cannot be resolved by traditionally trained doctors and specialists often are referred to psychologists for treatment. Yet when these patients begin a yeast-control diet and lifestyle, they respond splendidly, and their symptoms clear up. Even if Dr. Crook's yeast questionnaire does not prove conclusively that you have candidiasis, when you start the Body Ecology Diet, we guarantee that your health will improve and your symptoms will start disappearing.

Where Candida Grows

Candida grows in your intestines. According to antibody studies done at the Atkins Center, a yeast or fungal infection is involved in more than 80 percent of all cases of Crohn's disease and colitis.

When the immune system is weak, candida easily overruns the intestinal tract and the vagina, sinuses, and surfaces of the tongue. It also can burrow deeper into various organs. A carpet-like mass will wrap around the spinal cord and the nerves and often accumulates at the base of the brain. It can mass around the heart and liver, and it can affect the reproductive organs, even causing endometriosis in women.

Candida grows in your blood and is then called a systemic infection. The fungus (yeast) thrive on your own nutrients (minerals, proteins, and fats). This creates further deficiencies, especially of minerals (iron, selenium, zinc, etc.). Without minerals, your blood remains in an acidic condition.

The most important organs for creating energy are your adrenals and thyroid. They both need an ongoing steady supply of minerals. When mineral levels are low, you have very little energy. Feeling exhausted, you then crave carbohydrates for short-term energy. More minerals are called from various places (especially your bones and teeth) to keep a level of balance in your bloodstream. As your body continues to become even more acidic, the yeast infection escalates and can even become acute. Viral infections and cancer also grow and expand in this acidic condition.

Candida floods your body with toxic by-products called *acetaldehyde*, *gliotoxins*, and *mannan*. Acetaldehyde is the compound that produces the symptoms of an alcohol hangover. This serious toxin poisons tissues; is not easily eliminated; and accumulates in your brain, spinal cord, and muscles. (Remember that your heart and intestines are muscles.) You can now understand your symptoms of brain fog, muscle weakness, and even pain. Gliotoxins generate free radicals. They are very toxic to the immune system and destroy white blood cells that fight infections. This is why anyone with candida will suffer from frequent infections and why it is so difficult to conquer a yeast infection. Mannan also has a significant immunosuppressive effect.

The goal of the Body Ecology Diet is not to eliminate yeast from the body completely—this is impossible. It can live as an innocuous organism within our bodies. Instead, the goal is to conquer the runaway, pathogenic candida infection and bring the body back to a state of health where a strong immune system prevails.

Our next step is to investigate the basic principles of the Body Ecology system of health and healing.

❧

Notes

[3] Lorenzani, 1986.

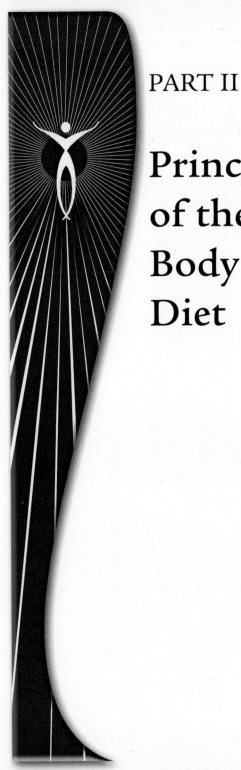

PART II

Principles of the Body Ecology Diet

Chapter 5

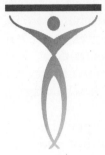

The Principle of Expansion and Contraction

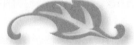

For more than 5,000 years Eastern philosophers have been using the extraordinary principle of yin/yang to explain how the universe works. In healing, as in all aspects of life, this simple, accurate universal law provides some answers to apparently mysterious conditions such as cancer, chronic fatigue syndrome, and candidiasis. The idea of mastering yin/yang is often overwhelming and could require a lifetime of study. To simplify matters, we are extracting the aspects of yin/yang that most apply to foods and healing. We call this the *expansion/contraction principle*. It stems from observations of natural phenomena. If mastering it at first seems a little complicated, relax—this principle is built right into the Body Ecology Diet. We present it here so you can obtain a basic understanding of how it works.

Ancient philosophers and healers observed that there are opposing forces in nature always seeking a balance. These opposing forces are not simply forces against one another, but are actually two parts of one whole. For example, male and female appear to be opposites, yet they really are extremes along the continuum of sexuality. "Maleness" is understood more clearly when compared with "femaleness." Left is better understood in relation to right. Up helps explain what down is.

While these forces appear to be opposites or even antagonistic forces, they really are complementary. For example, left complements right, since knowledge of left and right allows us to navigate and explore. Most of us would agree that male complements female, and vice versa.

When you combine any two complementary opposites, you can arrive at an ideal or a balance. For example, hot and cold create warmth.

The expansion/contraction principle is useful in understanding energy or *Ki* (life force within our bodies). Contracting energy or Ki is *stored* energy, while expanding energy is *released* energy. Contracting energy is *closed* and *tight*, while expanding energy is *open, relaxed*, and *active*. Expanding energy has a *fiery* nature, while contracting energy is like the nature of *water* . . . yielding, accepting, but persistent. The contracting force is soft, dark, surrendering, and intuitive in nature. Expansion indicates strength; brightness; and intense, forceful, potent energy (as in the energy of the sun).

It might be useful to point out here that extremes of contraction or expansion Ki are not ideal energy states when we are looking at the energy of the body. The ideal is the balance or midpoint of the two—when we feel calmly centered and truly strong.

Illness, therefore, is either extremely constrictive . . . closed and tightened energy; or extremely expansive . . . kinetic, nervous, uncomfortably intense energy. Candida itself is a rapidly growing, expanding fungus that thrives in the impure, dark, moist, contracted areas of the body.

To heal this condition we must stop the growth of this aggressive fungus by withholding the food it needs—and simultaneously change the imbalanced, weakened state of the immune system to a positive, energetic one. Eating appropriate foods is vital, because foods, too, are classified according to the expansion/contraction principle.

How the Expansion/Contraction Principle Affects the Foods We Eat

Some foods, such as salt, cause a contraction phenomenon within the body. Salt induces contraction of the cellular fluids. Too much salt can cause dehydration or extreme loss of bodily fluid. When we eat it, especially too much of it, we become thirsty. You have probably experienced this at a movie theater, if you have eaten the usual overly salted popcorn and become very thirsty.

Foods with salt inside them, such as animal foods[4] and cheese, also produce a contracting effect. Therefore, beef, pork, lamb, poultry, eggs, and fish are contracting foods. When we eat them, we feel more uptight or closed. A diet high in these foods can cause constipation.

Some foods, such as sugar, cause expansion to take place within the body. The bloodstream quickly absorbs sugar and produces energy. If you notice that you're feeling too contracted, you also might observe that you're beginning to crave something expansive (with sugar in it) to help you relax or feel more open. All foods with sugar in them (fruits, most dairy products, sweetened pastries, and candy) are expanding foods.

The Body Ecology Diet will teach you how to balance the foods you eat. Some foods are naturally balanced, and you'll want to eat them often. Please study the expansion/contraction chart on the following page carefully before reading on.

Besides sugar, note that alcohol, coffee, and drugs have an expanding effect. When consumed in excess, they cause too much expansion, and you can feel "spaced-out," confused, and unfocused.

Since a healthy body always strives toward balance, too much expanding food creates a craving for contracting food, and vice versa. For example, if you eat too much salt or animal food, you will crave sweets to make a balance. Eating this way puts your body on an undesirable seesaw. It's best to eat foods in the middle of the expansion/contraction spectrum, and when you do eat slightly toward one end or the other, choose foods that make a balance within the same meal. The Body Ecology Diet menus do this.

Remember that candidiasis is an expanding, rapidly growing condition within your body. To make a balance using the

FIGURE 2

The Expansion/Contraction Continuum

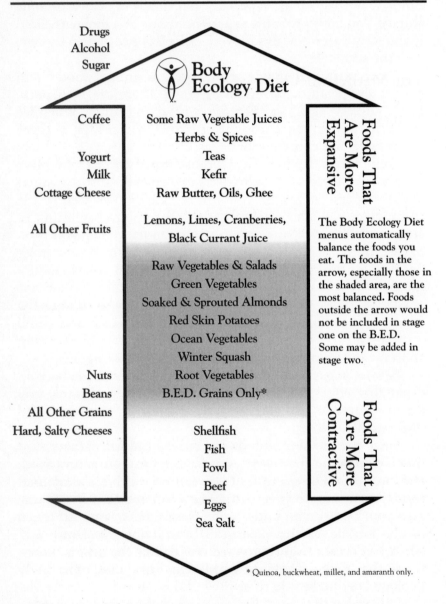

Drugs
Alcohol
Sugar

Body
Ecology Diet

Coffee

Some Raw Vegetable Juices

Herbs & Spices

Yogurt

Teas

Milk

Kefir

Cottage Cheese

Raw Butter, Oils, Ghee

All Other Fruits

Lemons, Limes, Cranberries,
Black Currant Juice

Foods That Are More Expansive

Raw Vegetables & Salads
Green Vegetables
Soaked & Sprouted Almonds
Red Skin Potatoes
Ocean Vegetables
Winter Squash

The Body Ecology Diet menus automatically balance the foods you eat. The foods in the arrow, especially those in the shaded area, are the most balanced. Foods outside the arrow would not be included in stage one on the B.E.D. Some may be added in stage two.

Nuts
Beans
All Other Grains
Hard, Salty Cheeses

Root Vegetables
B.E.D. Grains Only*

Foods That Are More Contractive

Shellfish
Fish
Fowl
Beef
Eggs
Sea Salt

* Quinoa, buckwheat, millet, and amaranth only.

appropriate foods, you should eat those foods that are slightly more contracting at first. And to strengthen a weak immune system, you need to eat more from the balanced center of the Expansion/Contraction Continuum. For example, at first you should eat more eggs (contracting) than you might normally. But always accompany them with vegetables (balanced). As your health improves, eat a larger percentage of your meals from the center of the chart (shaded area).

The Medicinal Value of Sea Salt

Salt is the most contracting food, but its role has been completely misunderstood. The ordinary table salt that most of us eat is too refined; it lacks the minerals we need and has harmful effects on the body. High-quality sea salt, however, is essential to life and has medicinal value in our diet.

For example, sea salt balances the expanding nature of butter and oils used in the Body Ecology Diet.

Why We Crave Sweets

Humans are contracted beings (we belong to the animal kingdom), so it is our nature to seek sweet, expanding tastes in an effort to balance the contraction. Newborn babies (tiny, contracted beings) thrive on breast milk, because it is sweet and watery; it is expanding.

Stress causes the body to contract. This too explains why we often crave expanding foods such as candy, alcohol, and even tobacco, because in our fast-paced world, we are usually under great stress.

The Body Ecology Diet satisfies this need with a naturally sweet herb, stevia. The sweet vegetables such as onions, carrots, and butternut squash also satisfy it. We use them abundantly in our recipes. The sour taste of our fermented foods negates the desire for sweets. You will feel well nourished and no longer crave foods containing sugars. Without refined carbs you will now lose weight, postpone aging, and reduce the susceptibility to diseases. If you are a parent feeling guilty about your child's constant craving for sugar, you'll find the solution in this book.

More on What to Eat

Whenever you eat contracting foods, it is vital to balance them with expanding foods that promote health. Since fruit is not on The Diet (and substances such as coffee, alcohol, and sugars inhibit healing), that leaves land and ocean vegetables, high-quality oil, butter, ghee, and simple herbs. These are excellent, healing foods, which contain all of nature's vitamins and minerals. The Body Ecology Diet recipes will teach you how to prepare many vegetables in ways you may never have known before, ways that will heal you.

Fish is the preferred animal food on The Diet. Among the contracting foods, fish ranks closest to the desirable balanced area (or shaded center area) of the expansion/contraction spectrum. Cold-water fish, such as tuna, salmon, and halibut, are the healthiest to eat; **avoid warm-water fish, such as orange roughy, because of the preservatives used when they are caught.**

In Summary

The foods listed within the shaded area of Figure 2, the Expansion/Contraction Continuum, provide the most healing energy for your body. Make them the main part of your diet, and when you eat outside the shaded area, make sure you balance your meals.

This does not mean you will never again eat foods outside the arrow. Indeed, once you have conquered your candidiasis and restored your immune system to health, you will be able to slowly reintroduce other healthy foods into your diet, foods such as beans, grains, nuts, and fruits. But while you are ridding your body of candidiasis, stick with the recommended foods; your reward will be extraordinary health and well-being.

ॐ

Notes

[4] The blood of animals is salty.

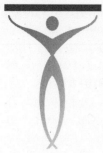

Chapter 6

The Principle of Acid and Alkaline

Just as our normal body temperature is 98.6 degrees F, there are other measures of a normal condition or homeostasis within the body. The levels of sugar, oxygen, and carbon dioxide in the blood must all be stable; and the pH (the balance between acid and alkaline) of the bodily fluids, including the blood, should be 7.4, slightly alkaline.

Knowledge of how to keep your blood in a slightly alkaline condition is vital to restoring your health. An imbalance toward too much acidity allows yeast, viruses, rebellious (cancer) cells, and various other parasites to thrive. Acidity also leads to conditions such as chronic fatigue, arthritis, and allergies.

The typical American diet is high in foods that cause our bodies to become acidic. It is no wonder, then, that these serious conditions are becoming more prevalent. If you have an acidic condition from eating an acid-forming diet, your body is constantly trying to return to a more balanced state by calling on your stored reserves of alkaline minerals: sodium, calcium, potassium, and magnesium. If you continue eating foods that are highly acid-forming, you deplete even more alkaline minerals from your body, creating a mineral deficiency that becomes severe over time.

The Simple, Obvious Solution

To overcome an acidic condition, eat alkaline-forming foods. But with candidiasis, we can eat only those alkaline-forming foods that do not feed yeast or parasites but that do rebuild the immune system. There are ten categories of alkaline-forming foods that satisfy these requirements.

Alkaline-Forming Foods You *Can* Eat:

- Most land vegetables
- Ocean vegetables (see Chapter 12)
- Millet, quinoa (pronounced "keen-wah"), and amaranth (available in health-food stores; see Chapter 12)
- Sea salt (good quality)
- Herbs and herb teas (organically grown; see Shopping List in Appendix A)
- Seeds (except sesame)
- Mineral water (sparkling and plain)
- Lemons; limes; berries; and sour, unsweetened juices from pomegranates, unsweetened cranberries, and black currants
- Raw apple cider vinegar
- Cultured vegetables and probiotic liquids (see Chapter 14)
- Milk kefir—if dairy works for you (see Chapter 15)
- Soaked and sprouted almonds[5]

Alkaline-Forming Foods Not on the Diet:

All other fruits.

Fruits create an alkaline condition when metabolized and are usually very good for us. However, when you have immune-system disorders, they are too high in sugar, and they feed yeast and other parasites.

Are Acid-Forming Foods Bad?

No. On the contrary, some acid-forming foods are necessary because of their nutritional value and for proper pH balance. The ideal acid-forming to alkaline-forming ratio by volume for any given meal should be:

Approximately 20% of the foods on your plate should be acid-forming, and approximately 80% should be alkaline-forming.

For more information on how to create the 80/20 balance, see Chapter 10 and Figure 7.

Acid-Forming Foods You *Can* Eat:

- Animal foods, such as beef, poultry, eggs, fish, and shellfish

- Buckwheat

- Organic, unrefined oils

- Stevia—liquid concentrate and white powder

Acid-Forming Foods You Should *Not* Eat:

Highly acid-forming foods not on The Diet include: sugar, candy, soft drinks, flour products, beans, soybean products and tofu, nuts (except almonds) and nut butters, wine, beer, saccharin, NutraSweet, alcohol, and commercial refined vinegar. Since all processed foods with preservatives and chemicals are acid-forming, please avoid them.

Examples of Balanced Meals Using the 20%/80% Acid/Alkaline Rule:

Example 1

- (20%) Softly scrambled eggs (1 whole + 2 yolks) . . .

- (80%) . . . with sautéed kale and onions and cultured vegetables
  Green tea sweetened with stevia if desired
  4 oz. young coconut kefir

Example 2
- (20%) A B.E.D. grain . . .

- (80%) . . . with sautéed onion, carrots, and peas
  Cultured vegetables
  4 oz. young coconut kefir
  Creamy broccoli soup
  Leafy green salad with salad dressing
  (using unrefined oils)

Example 3
- (20%) Grilled salmon . . .

- (80%) . . . with green beans with garlic
  Leeks and yellow squash sautéed with oregano and
  cultured vegetables

Can I Eat an All-Alkaline-Forming Meal?

Yes. Absolutely. All-alkaline-forming meals heal and balance. They are especially recommended for the first three days of The Diet to quickly restore the body to a more normal condition. We also recommend an all-alkaline meal whenever you are cleansing (see Chapter 8).

An example of such a meal would be:

Broccoli with Fresh Fennel Soup (see recipe in Part VII), cultured veggies, a medley of sautéed vegetables (onion, garlic, carrot, zucchini, and yellow squash), and a salad with the Body Ecology Diet Salad Dressing.

Do Any Foods Belong to a Neutral Group?

Yes, raw butter and ghee have a neutral pH balance.

What Else Causes Acidity?

Acidity in the blood/body fluids can be due to:
- Constipation.
- A deficiency of minerals (calcium, magnesium, potassium, sodium, etc.).

- Liver and/or kidney weakness.

- Overconsumption of protein from animal foods (see Chapter 10).

- Improper food combining (you'll read more about this soon).

- Overeating. People with body-ecology imbalances almost always overeat. They can't seem to satisfy their cravings, especially for sugar, bread, dairy, and fruit. This is partly because of the insatiable appetite of the yeast. Also, the lack of an inner ecosystem to help us properly digest food causes us to have nutritional deficiencies . . . some quite severe. So the body is desperately signaling us to feed it *real* food.

- Drug use (both medicinal and recreational). This stimulates the organs, releasing hormones and increasing the blood sugar. Taking drugs has the same negative effect as eating sugar. The body needs a large amount of minerals to return to balance.

- Exercise. This makes the blood acidic, but when you breathe deeply and rapidly as you exercise, your body releases carbon dioxide, and the blood then becomes more alkaline.

- Stress.

- Negative emotions, such as anger, resentment, guilt, and fear.

- Fatigue caused by stress.

Excess blood acidity weakens the respiratory system, resulting in less breathing, less oxygen inhaled, and, therefore, less oxygen available to your cells. This leads to further fatigue. No wonder that exhaustion is a common symptom of candidiasis, chronic fatigue, AIDS, and cancer. That's why we strongly recommend deep breathing and aerobic exercise to get more oxygen into your system.

If you feel that you are forgetful, spacey, or constantly disorganized, it could be because an acidic blood condition causes a lack of mental clarity. An alkaline body contributes to clear thinking and precise action.

FIGURE 3

Acid/Alkaline Foods

What's on the Body Ecology Diet Menu	**Acid-forming foods you can eat:**
	Animal foods (i.e., beef, poultry, eggs, fish, and shellfish)
	Buckwheat
	Organic, unrefined oils
	Stevia (an herb)
	
	Alkaline-forming foods you can eat:
	Land vegetables (most)
	Ocean vegetables
	Millet, quinoa, and amaranth
	Sea salt
	Herbs and herb teas
	Seeds (except sesame)
	Mineral water (plain or sparkling)
	Lemons, limes, unsweetened cranberries, and black currants
	Cultured foods
	    Raw organic apple cider vinegar
	    Raw cultured vegetables
	    Kefir (see Chapter 15)
	Soaked and sprouted almonds
	
	Neutral foods:
	Butter
	Ghee

What's Not on the Menu	**Acid-forming foods:** Sugar, candy, soft drinks Flour products Beans, soybean products, and tofu Nuts and nut butters Wine, beer, alcohol Saccharin, NutraSweet, Equal Commercial refined vinegar **Alkaline-forming foods:** Fruits (except those listed above)

When cells live too long in an acidic condition, they adapt to it by mutating and becoming malignant. Long-term acidic conditions in our bodies provide perfect environments for cancer and autoimmune diseases like AIDS to flourish. Most people with these disorders also have candidiasis.

Don't feel you have to master the science of acid/alkaline in order to get well. Yes, it takes some reading, study, and practice to feel comfortable with it, but the Body Ecology Diet has the acid/alkaline principle built right into it (see Figure 3 on facing page). Once you become familiar with all the elements of The Diet and learn the wonderful variety of foods available to you, you will soon be incorporating this principle easily into your menu planning.

⁂

Notes

[5] Almonds, while alkaline, are usually difficult to digest because of an enzyme-inhibiting substance contained in their brown coating. Soaking and sprouting removes this inhibitor. Almond butter is too high in oil for those of us with congested livers. (See Chapter 21.) All other nuts are acid-forming and are best avoided until your inner ecosystem is recolonized and your digestion improves.

Chapter 7

The Principle of Uniqueness

We humans share many features, but underneath, we all have distinct needs, different dreams, and changing situations.

This applies to our health, too. Our bodies change constantly. They change with the seasons, with the temperature, with where we live, with our age, with our mood. This means that we need different ways to stay healthy depending on all the variables that affect our daily lives.

We also live in a world where we constantly make choices from an overwhelming stream of information. All this freedom is wonderful, but it often comes with confusion about the "right" path, or the truth, or the best solution to our individual situations.

In this chapter we dispel some of the confusion you may be experiencing as you struggle to find what works for you. We offer insight into several of the most popular diets you might have read about or even tried for a while. We show you how the B.E.D. principles and foods synthesize the best of each of these, yet go even further to help you heal. Then you can make an informed choice and take action, always knowing you can change your path as your needs change, to find what's right for you. When you try a new way of eating, it's vital to observe your body's reactions and calmly assess whether this new path is bringing you back toward balance.

The Missing Link in Well-Known Diets

Each of the diets we discuss below teaches a portion of the "truth" that you may find useful for your own healing, but all are missing a critical element for optimal health. That element is the B.E.D. focus on the inner ecosystem, and the necessity of bringing it into balance. The blood type regimen, where you eat foods and even exercise according to your blood type, comes the closest to honoring the uniqueness of people, but it, like all the others, does not have an understanding of candidiasis and a compromised immune system. Yet, it has so much to offer that we devote an entire chapter to how it can help you, later in this book.

The High-Protein Diet

Perhaps the most popular of these alternative diets is the high-protein/low-carbohydrate system, attributed to Dr. Robert Atkins, and now appearing in many variations. Many people lose a lot of weight and feel very good when they start this diet. The carbohydrates that many of us consume to excess cause wild fluctuations in blood sugar and hormone levels, lead to storage of fat, create an acidic blood condition, and feed yeast. Eliminating them is essential. This diet also does a fair job of food combining, which helps people lose weight, eliminate bloating, and feel better (see Chapter 9).

Friendly bacteria and yeast must be present in the intestines to convert toxic by-products from the protein back into useful amino acids. If this does not occur, the intestines become foul and polluted. This contaminates your entire body. Over the long run, as the years go by, eating large amounts of animal protein two to three times a day puts a heavy burden on your liver, kidney, heart, and intestines.

The B.E.D. allows the animal proteins best for your blood type. We suggest you eat your protein meals between 11 A.M. and 2 P.M. if possible and strongly recommend taking digestive enzymes (see Chapte 12). Keep protein to about 20% of your meal, eat it with plenty of land and ocean vegetables, and very important, add friendly bacteria from cultured foods since they are essential to protein digestion.

We also suggest you obtain protein from vegetarian sources such as algae, soaked seeds and almonds, and later from fermented soy (miso) and milk kefir (if you digest casein). As your digestion improves, you can eat soaked and sprouted beans (raw or cooked) with vegetables (raw, cooked, and cultured).

High-protein diets lack adequate fiber. On the B.E.D., fiber comes in part from high-protein seed-like grains that comprise an important aspect of The Diet and contribute to a healthy inner ecosystem.

The Raw Foods Diet

Developed by Ann Wigmore many years ago, this diet results in a rapid elimination of toxins, with an emphasis on cleansing the liver and colon. It is very beneficial for people with cancer who have to detoxify quickly in order to save their lives. Eating raw foods is essential if you are struggling with an active viral condition such as full-blown AIDS, or a herpes outbreak. But when the viral infection is dormant, you must have a diet that is more strengthening.

You see, viruses are present in the blood of most people, and certainly in those with a yeast condition. A healthy immune system keeps these viruses dormant and under control. But as you know from reading Chapter 6, when the body becomes too acidic, the viruses seize the opportunity to thrive, and you have an outbreak. When viral infections become active like this, there is always a low-grade internal "fever." So you need to eat raw foods, which "cool" the body.

Thus, you could manage any viral condition by eating the right foods at the appropriate time, and carefully monitoring your body's response. While the virus is inactive, nourish and strengthen your body with ample "warming" (cooked) and some raw and cultured foods. When the virus becomes active, cool and cleanse your body with raw foods. Ideally, a raw foods diet works best during hot weather and while living in a warm climate. If you do a little research, you'll note that all the major advocates of the raw foods movement have centers in climates such as Florida, Arizona, California, or Puerto Rico.

Many people who practice the raw foods diet often have a poor understanding of the value of organic, unrefined fats and oils—important B.E.D. foods. The raw foods diet usually violates food-combining rules and allows too many fruits and sweet desserts made from fruits and nuts. On the other hand, you'll find some great recipes for making patés and dehydrated "crackers" from seeds, nuts, and vegetables. Just don't overdo these. Nuts are rich in arginine, an amino acid that triggers viral outbreaks, and also oxalates. Oxalate-rich foods often are not tolerated when there is gut dysbiosis. If your energy suddenly drops after eating them, it's a clue they are not good for you.

If you decide to try the B.E.D. version of a raw foods diet, be sure to avoid fruit, wheat grass, Rejuvelac, and Braggs Amino Acids. They will intensify your yeast problem.

The Macrobiotic Diet

I (Donna) am deeply grateful for my macrobiotic training. While studying this system of healing, I learned many of the medicinal benefits of the Japanese way of eating. This includes a variety of delicious yet therapeutic foods such as the root vegetables daikon and burdock. A macrobiotic meal always includes a dark green leafy vegetable and uses excellent immune-strengthening foods like shiitake mushrooms and miso soup.

Unfortunately, many macrobiotic-acceptable foods contribute to yeast overgrowth. Even though a variety of grains are allowed, macrobiotic dieters eat mostly brown rice. The portions of grain are too large, often as much as 70% of your plate. When you read more about the 80/20 principle in Chapter 10, you will learn that the majority of your plate should be vegetables and the remainder a B.E.D. grain-like seed or a protein. Macrobiotics would be a much healthier diet if it balanced all the cooked foods with raw cultured vegetables, a mainstay of the B.E.D. Some animal protein is allowed on this diet, but most macrobiotic eaters get their protein from tofu, tempeh, and miso soup, which the B.E.D. does not recommend in the first stages of healing. Also, these soy products are not the best source of protein for those with blood type B.

Macrobiotics is a fairly rigid way of eating and a diet that lacks joy. It frowns upon herbs and spices, which results in bland tastes and inhibits the medicinal value of these flavorings. In addition, the heavy use of salt causes a sort of rigidity. Remember, salt is the most contracting food on the Expansion/Contraction Continuum.

The Vegetarian Diet

The Body Ecology Diet can easily work well if you are not a strict vegan and are willing to eat some eggs. In time as your digestion becomes stronger, kefir made from goat, sheep, or cow milk could be a good vegetarian protein as well (but not vegan). Fermented soybean foods like natto, tempeh, and miso will provide you with vegan protein. Fermented spirulina and other algae in products like Body Ecology's Vitality SuperGreen or our Potent Proteins enhance a vegan diet. Healing always requires additional protein. Good news: the B.E.D. "grains," really seeds, are high in protein. So are the nuts (soaked almonds) and seeds (pumpkin, flax, sunflower) allowed on The Diet. Remember, you can add soaked and sprouted beans later. They should always be cooked. Dark green leafy vegetables have protein, too.

Minerals are essential for the assimilation of protein, yet without the friendly flora in the intestines to "hold on to" them, they are not retained. Microflora colonizing the small intestine work hard to create mineral-rich blood for you. In addition, yeast and fungus subtract protein and minerals from the body as they feed themselves. So if you lack an abundant inner ecosystem, you are most likely deficient in both these important elements.

Even if you have been a vegetarian for years, please consider adding some fresh fish even temporarily as you begin The Diet. It has medicinal, grounding, and strengthening properties. Digestive enzymes and lots of cultured vegetables will help ensure you digest the fish easily.

You Are the Creator of Your Own Body

As the seasons of the year move from hot to cold and back, and as your body's ever-changing condition and nutritional requirements shift, your food choices will, too. You'll have the freedom to move between raw foods (when you want to cool and cleanse your body and/or rest the liver) and steamed, simmered, broiled, and baked foods (when you need easily digested, warming foods). In the colder winter months, you'll enjoy more cooked meals plus a little more of the good organic, unrefined oils and sea salt. In the hottest days of summer, you'll use sea salt and these medicinal oils sparingly, if at all. You'll add the right percentage of animal foods (the ones that are best for your blood type) when you need grounding and strengthening (which for many people is every day). You'll obtain your much-needed minerals from ocean vegetables. And, with every meal, you will munch the most priceless of all the edibles, cultured foods, to build a magnificent inner ecosystem.

Are you still wondering why we have so many seemingly conflicting choices? Because, like a snowflake, each of us is uniquely special. We're given an abundance of solutions to care for our constantly changing bodies. The challenge is to know ourselves and seek the solution that is right for us at this moment in time. We can always turn within for guidance, and the appropriate course of action will reveal itself. Everything we need to be healthy and happy is available to us right now.

Chapter 8

The Principle of Cleansing

The principle of cleansing may be the most important of the seven principles that make up the Body Ecology Diet. Yet, initially, it is the most misunderstood and least trusted of them all. The earth we live on undergoes a constant cleansing and renewal process. All creatures, including humans, live according to the truly wondrous law of cleansing.

Cleansing allows our bodies to restore balance when the imbalance becomes too great and threatens our lives. Sadly, most of us have no understanding and no gratitude for this essential, life-saving process occurring within us. If you forget the other six principles on The Diet but begin to master this one, you will still be on your way to becoming well.

Cleansing is your body's natural way to get rid of waste or toxins, and it occurs daily in some form or another. Tears, urine, mucus, sweat—all are examples of body cleansing that we regard as very normal. But the body has other normal ways to eliminate harmful substances—giving us such disruptions as fevers, colds, and skin eruptions—and we have been taught that these are bad and need to be suppressed.

Nothing could be further from the truth.

The body is designed to rid itself naturally of toxins and waste, but when we take drugs, we drive these toxins deeper into our systems, and they further weaken vital organs. Eventually, the weakened organs have no energy to eliminate toxins and fight disease; they give up the fight, and the body succumbs to illness.

Look at Figure 4. The top diagram shows a series of peaks and valleys. The peaks represent the positive times when our bodies are rebuilding. We feel great and look great. The valleys are the times of cleansing when we ache or feel tired, feverish, or ill. In the first rebuilding/cleansing cycle, you see the ups and downs, but the overall trend is up: the chart of an increasingly healthy body that does not stop its cleansings. In the middle diagram, the overall trend or direction is down: the diagram of a body unable to fight off true disease, because it frequently takes medication and is not using the best weapons of healing— appropriate food, water, rest, and exercise.

We all have peaks and valleys in our health throughout our lives. The valleys are periods of cleansing we should be grateful for. After the cleansing is over, our bodies will be free of damaging toxins, and this leads to a lifetime of greater strength and health. *You cannot heal without cleansing.*

As you follow The Diet, ridding your body of accumulated toxins, you will have ups and downs—but you will see that, as the months pass, the overall direction will be up. Your symptoms may temporarily flare up, and sometimes you will think you are even "sicker" than before you started The Diet, but this is short-lived. It is often due to the die-off of the yeast. Yes, yeast secrete toxic substances when they are alive and create toxins when they are dying. Once these toxins have left your body, you will feel much stronger.

Also, when you eat healthier foods, your immune system becomes stronger and more yeast start to die. With The Diet, your body will start to have more energy, but with this newfound energy, your cells will begin to push out their toxins. Too many toxins flood into your bloodstream, and because your body can't eliminate them fast enough, your symptoms become worse. (See Chapter 18, on colon cleansing.) While we know it is difficult to do so, welcome these cleansings, because they mean you are getting well.

FIGURE 4

Ups and Downs of Cleansing

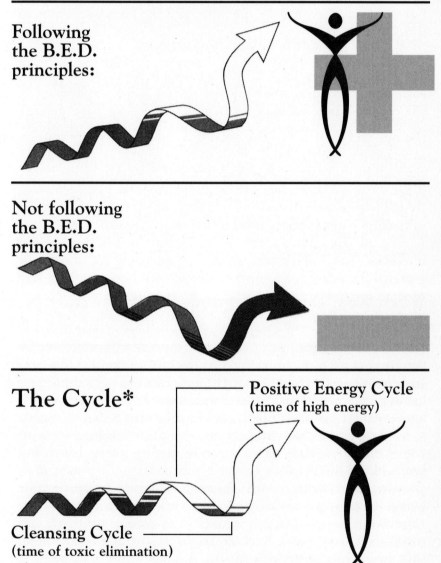

Following
the B.E.D.
principles:

Not following
the B.E.D.
principles:

The Cycle*

Positive Energy Cycle
(time of high energy)

Cleansing Cycle
(time of toxic elimination)

* The cycle will happen regardless of whether the individual is on the B.E.D. However, following the principles of The Diet will move an individual in a positive health direction.

Difference Between Cleansing and Disease

Cleansing is a continuing, step-by-step phenomenon. It is the natural force that drives impurities from the body: impurities resulting from the poor quality of our diets, our environment, and our emotional lives. Disease, on the other hand, often occurs when the body loses its ability to cleanse itself and gives up the struggle to remain pure.

The cleansing process is very simple: When the organs of elimination (lungs, liver, kidneys, colon) become overwhelmed with impurities and toxins, these toxins lodge somewhere in the cells, tissues, or muscles (usually where we have genetic weaknesses). In an attempt to maintain integrity, the body organizes a cleansing, forcing the toxins out in some disruptive form like fever, cold, flu, rashes, acne, or other "illness." If a cleansing is suppressed by a drug (such as an antibiotic or a cold medicine), the toxins are driven deeper into the body. Over time, the major organs give up a little of their fight to stay alive until, step by step, they give up altogether, becoming weakened and diseased.

When We Cleanse, Symptoms Get Worse . . . Temporarily

Your most significant period of cleansing will occur during your first three months, and especially during the first few days and weeks, on the Body Ecology Diet. This is a period of great healing. As we have just mentioned, you are offering your body high-quality, well-combined, healthy food that is easy to digest. It will respond by showing extensive signs of healing—only to you it may look and feel as if you're getting worse. Cleansing looks like a disturbance to the entire system. Compare it to cleaning your living room. When you decide to clean your living room, you start dusting, vacuuming, and cleaning the windows. The dirt and grime start to fly, you move furniture, throw things out—and if someone arrives during the middle of this, your living room looks awful. But when you're finished, it looks much better than before.

When your body starts cleansing, you may have a sore throat, skin eruptions, headaches, flu symptoms, aches and pains, depression, lethargy, increased fatigue, skin rashes, and vaginal itching and discharge. This is just evidence that your body is throwing out those accumulated toxins. This is known as the Herxheimer die-off reaction. As the yeast die off and exit through normal body channels, they release toxins that cause these symptoms. The greater the die-off, the more uncomfortable you may be. It's extremely important to remain strictly on The Diet during this time, to give yourself the maximum opportunity to heal. It's easy to get discouraged when you find yourself just as "sick" as before, but have faith that when this healing period ends, you definitely will feel stronger and better. A home enema or a visit to your colon therapist at the first sign of cleansing will greatly shorten and minimize any discomfort (see Chapter 18). When the cleansing ends, you will be free of symptoms that may have plagued you for years; you will be much stronger and healthier.

The Length of the Cleansing Process

It's different for everybody, and it depends on how long the toxins have been in your body and how deeply embedded they are. For some, it takes three months to a year to be symptom free; for many with severe candida imbalance, it may take longer, possibly up to three years. Most people feel a lot better after only two weeks on The Diet. You may be surprised to find yourself choosing to stay on the expanded version of the Body Ecology Diet (see Chapter 22), adding the foods you can tolerate, forever. The reward for such self-discipline will be clearly demonstrated in the quality of the way you live the rest of your life: as someone who experiences the full joy of a strong, healthy body and mind, with enough energy to do whatever you want.

Hints to Help You Stick with the Diet During Cleansing

- Eat all-alkaline meals, especially during the first three days on The Diet (see Chapter 6).

- Eat warming foods, such as vegetable soup.

- Don't overeat, because this diverts your energy from cleansing to digestion. An age-old remedy forgotten by our generation is to clean your colon at the first sign of a cleansing (see Chapter 18).

- If you crave sweets, satisfy that craving with the herb stevia. Use it in teas, or check out our recipes that use stevia.

- Get plenty of rest. Be kind to yourself. Let your body heal.

- Find someone to talk to who has already gone through this intensive initial cleansing, someone who will encourage you not to give up.

- Be patient. Cleansing occurs in incremental steps, just like the transition from darkness to daylight. You can't hurry it.

The Emotional Side of Cleansing and Healing

The impact of our thoughts and feelings on the body is well documented, and the new field of psychoneuroimmunology relates this to the health of the immune system. Through techniques such as visualization, affirmations, and even prayer, we can strengthen our immune systems and enhance the cleansing/healing process. If we try to heal our bodies but remain angry, stressed, or guilty in our minds, the healing will take longer and be more difficult. But if we can cleanse our minds of negative, impure thoughts and emotions, replacing them with joy, love, and trust, the physical cleansing and healing will be easier and more fulfilling.

As your physical body cleanses itself, you may feel inexplicably weepy, on edge, or angry. (Spring and fall are two natural times for cleansings.) Without warning, you may feel like lashing out at someone verbally or even physically. Or you might start crying about something seemingly small. This is all part of the elimination of stored-up emotional toxins connected to the physical toxins in your body—just know that these feelings are normal, and it's beneficial to release them in a safe environment.

It may help you to keep in mind that nature is constantly cleansing our environment with storms, hurricanes, tidal waves, floods, ice, and snow. Think about the aftereffects of a spring storm: doesn't the air seem fresh, clean, and pure?

HEALING HINTS: Take a few minutes once or several times each day to stop what you are doing, breathe deeply, and appreciate the good things about your life and surroundings. Seek the serenity and peace that are essential to good health and strength.

A Special Gift for Women

The monthly menstrual cycle offers women a special opportunity to cleanse. Not only does the uterus shed its lining during this normal process, but the entire body enters a cleansing mode. So to take advantage of this opportunity, treat yourself well. Rest a little more; plan quiet activities; and eat warm, alkaline-forming foods. This regular cleansing is one of the reasons women have traditionally outlived men. Men do not have this opportunity to cleanse as frequently.

The process of *pregnancy* and *childbirth* also allows women to cleanse. During birth, a tremendous amount of toxins— some built up over a longer period than the nine months of pregnancy— leave the body with the baby and the afterbirth. Afterward, especially if she is on the Body Ecology Diet, a woman can be even healthier: her skin color may be more porcelain-like, her chronic vaginitis gone. Sadly, many valuable nutrients also leave the mother's body unless she eats a nutrient-dense, probiotic diet. The B.E.D. is ideal. Unfortunately for her baby, many of her toxins are now concentrated in her newborn.

You Can Choose How Quickly You Want to Cleanse

The Body Ecology Diet works because it supports your body in doing what it was designed to do: cleanse. Cleansing equals healing. However, while you can't stop and never want to stop cleansings, you might like to know that you have some control over how quickly you cleanse.

When you begin conquering your immune-system disorder, you simply need to follow The Diet *strictly*, eating only the foods allowed and following the food-combining rules. Yeast will begin dying off immediately, and your body will begin sending the dead yeast out through the usual channels (into the bloodstream, then out via the urine, bowel movements, respiration, sweat, and, for women, through the vagina).

Remember, at first the yeast may be dying off faster than your body can handle; you may experience a variety of symptoms such as fatigue, spaciness, heaviness, depression, anger, and flu and cold symptoms. While this will clear up (usually within three to ten days), you can shorten the duration of the cleansing and minimize your discomfort by cleansing your colon with an enema or a colonic (see Chapter 18). It is not necessary to take candida-control products or "yeast fighters" sold in health-food stores until you are ready to go to a deeper level of cleansing. Initially they may cause too much die-off. These products can be useful later when you want to go to a deeper level of healing. For now, spend your money on the best-quality foods and colon hydrotherapy.

Don't be afraid to cleanse; expect it, even welcome it. If you find yourself cleansing so much that you cannot function, do what is recommended when you come down with a cold . . . cleanse the colon, rest, keep warm, and drink lots of fluids, such as hot water with lemon juice or warm teas.

How quickly do you want to cleanse? If you found yourself climbing a challenging mountain where everything you ever wanted was awaiting you at the top, how fast would you like to get there? Conquering this condition is like climbing a challenging mountain. You'll have to go step by step using special tools to make the job easier, but it's you who will decide how fast to go.

Toward a New Science

Thousands of years ago ancient Chinese healers knew the dangers of suppressing the body's natural healing process. Their work was to enhance the Ki or Chi (life force energy). Oriental medicine uses natural herbs to activate (not suppress) the energy of the cleansing organs so that they can do the job they were created to do. Medicines used by modern Western science today stop, close down, or interfere with the "pushing out" process of cleansing. Medical researchers need to do a 180-degree turnabout and look for ways to support our cleansing organs, not suppress and choke the life out of them. If we would keep our bodies as pure as the day we were born—enzyme- and oxygen-rich; inhabited abundantly with friendly bacteria; and rich in proteins, minerals, and essential fatty acids—we might be able to live for hundreds of years. We must develop a "New Medical Science" by tuning in to nature and learning from it instead of ignorantly and arrogantly fighting our natural healing process.

"Food is medicine" is an old Chinese saying. The Body Ecology Diet incorporates exactly the foods that heal immune-system disorders and weaves them into a delicious, nutritious diet plan.

But even eating the healthiest foods won't stop you from cleansing. Cleansings are nature's brilliant attempt to keep us healthy so we can enjoy a long, happy life. When we go against nature, we create unhappiness, disorder, and disease.

Our medical community must begin crossing natural healing methods with modern scientific technology, with an emphasis on wellness, prevention, and wholesome nutrition—rather than continuing to support the development of drugs that damage the immune system. Fortunately, many at the forefront of medicine already have.

Chapter 9

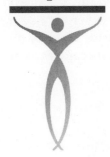

The Principle of Food Combining

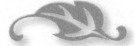

Food combining means what to eat with what. It's an important feature of the B.E.D. and one reason The Diet works while other anti-candida diets do not.

Even if you no longer eat foods that feed the yeast, the overgrowth of yeast in your system won't disappear if you are combining these foods improperly. To conquer candidiasis, it is essential to practice the principles of proper food combining. There are two reasons for this:

- Eating foods together that are not compatible in the stomach (see Figure 5 at the end of the chapter) causes poor digestion and leads to fermentation. This fermentation produces alcohol and sugars, and the yeast feed off these sugars and multiply rapidly, creating more toxins in the body.

- People with candidiasis have overly sensitive digestive tracts. Improper food combining further stresses the digestive tract and causes it to work even less efficiently.

By following the rules of proper food combining, you avoid fermentation in the digestive system. The healing process begins by allowing the overworked digestive tract to begin to function as it should, and a healthy digestive tract is an important first step toward the total renewal that restores your body's balanced ecology.

Benefits of Food Combining

- You'll feel better. You will be less bloated and will stop having symptoms such as gas and stomach gurgling.

- You'll have a system to guide your choice of foods, an approach that makes it easier to decide what to eat. You'll be better able to stick with The Diet.

- You'll never be overweight. In fact, you'll probably lose some weight. Properly combined food is assimilated better and allows the body to metabolize it better and avoid storing fat.

- You'll have more energy.

The Basics

Food combining can be summarized in three basic rules.

Rule #1:

Eat fruits alone and on an empty stomach.

Fruits encourage the growth of yeast in the body, so as you begin the Body Ecology Diet, the only fruits allowed are very sour ones like lemons, limes, and berries. Unsweetened juices from pomegranates, cranberries, and black currants are also allowed. These are acidic[6] or "sour" fruits. Low in sugar, they do not create yeast overgrowth. All other fruits are too sweet.

Fruits pass through the digestive system very quickly. They usually leave the stomach within 30 minutes and enter the small intestine, where they continue to be digested. But if you eat them with other foods (such as a protein or starch) that take three to five hours or more to digest, the fruit is held up and starts to ferment. This means poor assimilation of nutrients but, more important, it sets up a perfect environment for yeast overgrowth, as they feed off the sugar produced from the fermentation.

While it's best to eat fruit alone, proper food combining allows you to eat acidic or sour fruits with *protein fat* foods such as milk kefir, yogurt, or nuts and seeds. For example, you could combine strawberries, blueberries, or pomegranate juice with yogurt or milk kefir . . . or a handful of soaked and sprouted sunflower seeds.

As your health improves and you introduce more fruits, stay with the "sour" fruits, like grapefruit and kiwi. They are also low-sugar fruits and have enough of an acidic quality that they usually don't activate yeast symptoms. Remember, the sweeter fruits have too much sugar.

The only time your stomach is truly empty is when you wake up in the morning. So, that's the best time to eat fruit like blueberries. Sweet fruits in the morning weaken your adrenals. Please note that one of the most frequent mistakes is to introduce new foods, especially sweet foods, too soon, before your yeast infection is fully conquered and your body ecology is restored. If you do not have a body-ecology imbalance, sour fruit could be an ideal breakfast, because it contains a lot of water, which your system needs after being asleep without fluid all night. When you wake up, we highly recommend drinking a couple of glasses of water, because your body is dehydrated, before eating the sour fruit. Adding lemon juice to your second glass of water is an age-old way to stimulate the peristaltic action of your colon. A "probiotic juice" combining a sour juice (like black currant juice) with a probiotic drink (young coconut kefir or Body Ecology's Cocobiotic) adds beneficial bacteria to your digestive tract. Black currant juice (unsweetened) is used to stimulate the appetite and soothe upset stomachs. It is recommended for anemia, is rich in vitamin C, is a great antioxidant, and nourishes the adrenals. We love it, too, because only a few ounces will give you lots of energy.

One exception to this rule is lemons and animal protein. Lemon juice squeezed onto a piece of grilled salmon, for example, aids digestion and provides a nice expansion/contraction balance.

Rule #2:

Always eat protein with non-starchy and/or ocean vegetables.

When you eat animal-protein foods such as eggs, meat, poultry, and fish, your stomach must produce hydrochloric acid and an enzyme called pepsin to digest them. When you eat animal-protein foods such as eggs, meat, poultry, and fish, your stomach must produce hydrochloric acid and an enzyme called pepsin to digest them. While digestion of protein *begins* in your stomach, it continues breaking down and is assimilated once it reaches your small intestine. The carbohydrates and the fats eaten at that meal digest only when they reach it. The digestive enzymes produced by the small intestine are alkaline. When you eat a starchy food, such as a potato or rice, with a protein, like chicken, this creates too much work for your digestive tract and results in poor digestion, then fermentation, which creates sugars and a field day for the yeast.

Non-starchy vegetables and ocean vegetables are the most compatible foods to eat with protein meals. They require neither a strong alkaline nor a strong acid condition to digest properly. So by eating protein foods with non-starchy vegetables, you can achieve optimal digestion.

Recommended Non-starchy Vegetables

Asparagus	Celery root	Kohlrabi
Bamboo shoots	Chives	Lamb's-quarters
Beet greens	Collard greens	Leeks
Bok choy	Cucumber	Lettuces
Broccoli	Daikon	Mustard greens
Brussels sprouts	Dandelion greens	Okra
Burdock root	Endive	Onion
Cabbage	Escarole	Parsley
Carrots	Fennel	Radishes (red)
Cauliflower	Garlic	Red bell pepper
Celeriac	Green beans	Scallions
Celery	Jicama	Shallots
	Kale	

Spinach	Swiss chard	Watercress
Sprouts	Turnips	Zucchini
(except mung bean)	(and greens)	

Non-starchy vegetables go with just about everything. You can eat them with oil; butter; ghee; animal flesh; eggs; grains; starchy vegetables (like acorn squash and potatoes); lemons; limes; and raw sunflower, caraway, flax, or pumpkin seeds.

Menu Tips:

Combine:
- Fish with stir-fried or steamed vegetables.

- Chicken with a leafy green vegetable and an all-vegetable soup such as cream of cauliflower with dill.

- A large vegetable salad with protein (chilled salmon or sliced boiled egg) and dressing (oil free or from organic, unrefined oils).

- An onion, red pepper, and zucchini omelette or ocean vegetable omelette with steamed asparagus and garlic.

Rule #3:

Always eat grains, grain-like seeds, and starchy vegetables with non-starchy and/or ocean vegetables.

The grain-like seeds that are allowed on the Body Ecology Diet in stage one are amaranth, quinoa, buckwheat, and millet. Starchy vegetables include acorn and butternut squash, lima beans, English peas, corn (fresh), water chestnuts, artichokes and Jerusalem artichokes, and red skin[7] potatoes. Combine them with non-starchy vegetables or ocean vegetables for some delicious, filling meals.

Combine:
- Millet casserole, a steamed leafy green vegetable, and yellow squash and leeks sautéed in butter.

- Buckwheat/quinoa/millet croquettes topped with the Body Ecology Diet Gravy, steamed greens, and carrot-cauliflower soup.

- Dilled potato salad, watercress soup, and a leafy green salad with Body Ecology Diet Salad Dressing.

- Acorn squash stuffed with curried quinoa, broccoli with seasoned butter, and the sea vegetable hijiki with onions and carrots.

Fats and Seed Oils

There are many delicious fats and oils allowed on The Diet. The only oils we recommend are freshly pressed, organic, and *unrefined* oils (flax seed, evening primrose, borage seed, pumpkin seed, and walnut). Extra-virgin olive oil is also excellent, and you can use this oil generously. The fats you will want to eat include unrefined, organic coconut oil, butter,[8] and ghee.

Never combine a large amount of fat with a protein. Large amounts of fat, especially *refined* fats, delay the secretion of hydrochloric acid needed to digest the protein. An example of this is mayonnaise with tuna or chicken . . . creating the popular "tuna salad" (usually made into an even more poorly combined sandwich). Use a dressing made with one or more of the oils mentioned above or use an oil-free dressing to make tuna, egg, or chicken salads. (See recipes.)

Cooking Tips:

If you need a small amount of oil in your cooking to keep food from sticking to the pan, we recommend coconut oil, olive oil, butter, or ghee. You also might try using broth or even water to avoid the sticking.

Do not eat hydrogenated fats, such as margarine. The hydrogenation process changes the character of the oils used, making them poisonous.

Protein Fats

Avocado, olives, cheese, seeds, and nuts (except chestnuts and peanuts, which are starchy) belong to a category classified as "protein fats." These foods combine best with non-starchy and green vegetables, ocean vegetables, and acid fruits.

While cheese is not on stage one of The Diet, nuts and seeds are . . . as long as you can digest them. To make them more digestible, always soak them at least eight hours before eating. They can also be soaked, then dehydrated at a low temperature; and/or soaked and pureed into a paté. Avocados can be eaten if they work in your unique body, but olives are best avoided, as they often contain mold. Avocados and olives are really fruits and only combine well with non-starchy vegetables, ocean vegetables, and *acid* fruits, as we've just mentioned.

Dairy

Dairy foods also belong to the category of protein fats. Most milk products contain milk sugar (lactose) that feeds yeast, so avoid them on stage one of The Diet. These foods also contain casein, the main protein in dairy products (except human breast milk, which has more whey protein than casein). In the beginning, you may have a permeable, leaky gut; and the casein will enter your bloodstream and cause allergic-like symptoms that can be very obvious or very subtle.

Fermented, homemade milk kefir (see Chapter 15) has much less lactose, and the casein is pre-digested. Every body is unique, of course, but dairy products may become a nourishing food for you in stage two of The Diet. If so, introduce them slowly, and only after your gut lining has healed and your inner ecosystem is restored. For some, dairy foods should be avoided forever. If and when you do eat them, combine dairy foods with acidic fruits,[9] seeds and nuts, and non-starchy vegetables (especially raw, leafy greens). For example, create a milk kefir salad dressing using lemon juice, avocado, Hawaiian sea salt, and fresh herbs and toss into mixed field greens. You could also sprinkle in some soaked and sprouted pumpkin seeds.

Dried Beans, Peas, and Soybeans

These foods are not on stage one of The Diet, so you won't be eating them initially. They are mostly starch, with some protein, so you can see why they are difficult to digest and cause gas. When your digestive tract becomes stronger, you may be able to introduce them and combine them safely with non-starchy green vegetables and ocean vegetables. For example, try anasazi beans cooked with onion and garlic, served with sautéed carrots, daikon, and steamed greens or a raw salad. Soybeans should be fermented. Miso, natto, and wheat-free low-sodium tamari are recommended in stage two of The Diet but can even be eaten by many in stage one. These are good choices of protein for vegans and vegetarians, and they are easy to digest. Tempeh does not feed yeast but causes embarrassing gas for many.

Sugar, Honey, Molasses, etc.

The Body Ecology Diet is sugar free because sugars feed yeast. For years we have used stevia liquid concentrate to satisfy our natural desire for sweet-tasting foods and beverages. In November 2007, Body Ecology introduced a new non-caloric sweeter called Lakanto to the American market. See Part VII for an update on Lakanto.

Sugars should be eaten alone; they don't combine with anything! That's why you can get gas from cookies, since they combine starches, fruits, and sugars. Never eat sugar if you want to remain healthy and free of yeast. And if you give your taste buds a chance to adjust to the new sweet taste of stevia and Lakanto, you may never want sugar again anyway.

Your Weight

Proper food combining automatically results in weight loss. Some people can easily lose up to ten pounds during the first two weeks after they start The Diet. This is all very normal—don't worry if you lose more weight than you want. Within three months, or perhaps even sooner, you will find that you've reached an ideal weight for your frame. If you're already thin, you will still lose some bloating; the scales may stay the same, but you'll look different.

When you practice the rules of proper food combining, you may feel hungrier than usual. Again, this is because you'll have no "bloated" or full feeling after meals. So just eat smaller amounts more often! It's fine to have four to five smaller meals throughout the day. As long as your food is properly

FIGURE 5

B.E.D. Food-Combining Chart

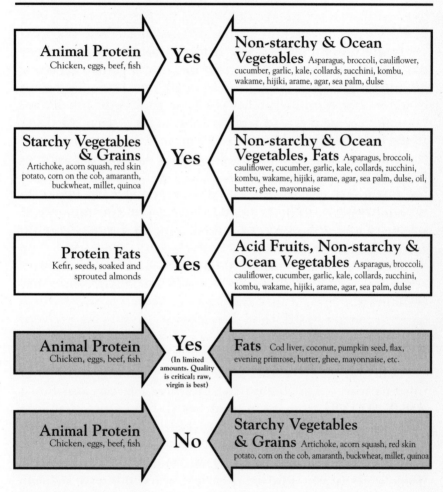

NOTES: All fruits should be eaten alone (30 minutes before or 3 hours after eating) with exception of the acid fruits, which may be eaten with protein fats. Only very sour acid fruits are on the B.E.D. (lemons, limes, cranberries, and black currant juice).
SUGAR–Not on B.E.D. but should be eaten alone (30 minutes before or 3 hours after eating). Does not combine well with any other foods.
DAIRY–Not on B.E.D. If introduced later, ferment and eat alone (30 minutes before or 3 hours after eating) or with raw salads, acid fruits, or seeds and nuts.
PROTEIN STARCHES–Dried peas, soybeans, and beans are not initially on B.E.D. If introduced later, they should then be eaten with non-starchy vegetables and cultured veggies.

combined, you can eat as often as you need to and not worry about gaining weight. Just allow time for a meal that contains protein to digest (about three hours) before switching to a meal with grain-like seeds.

Water

Drink water alone. Ideally, drink at least eight glasses per day, but not with meals, since it dilutes your digestive enzymes. When you get up in the morning, drink two 12-ounce glasses of water almost immediately to hydrate your body. It will have become very dehydrated from a long night's sleep. At other times, drink no closer than 10 to 15 minutes before a meal, and then wait again an hour or longer after you eat. Drink water at room or body temperature—ice-cold water shocks the system too much. Try to have at least half your daily water intake by mid-morning; it really revitalizes your system. Having a cup of warm tea and/or a bowl of soup adds liquid during the meal. This aids digestion, but soups and tea are foods. And even though they contain water, they are not as hydrating as water and should not be counted as one of your eight glasses of water each day.

Additional Resources

Many books are available on food combining, and lots of information is available on the Internet. You can also buy a wallet-size card from your local health-food store that lists different food groups and tells you which foods combine well.

Don't let all this confuse you. It takes a bit of practice, but soon it becomes second nature, and you'll automatically know what foods to eat together. Proper food combining is a key part of the Body Ecology Diet, and mastering it will reward you with better health.

Notes

[6] Not to be confused with the acid/alkaline principle. For a list of acidic fruits, see page 211.

[7] Red skin potatoes have less sugar than other varieties and do not feed yeast.

[8] Raw butter is best if available. To make your own raw cultured butter, see page 104.

[9] Black currant juice and cranberry juice are delicious in kefir. Sweeten with Body Ecology's stevia liquid concentrate.

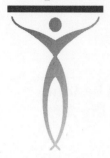

Chapter 10

The Principle of 80/20

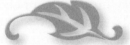

When you have candidiasis or other immune-system diseases, it is essential that the food you eat be properly assimilated and then eliminated. A healthy digestive tract can do this. But many people weaken their digestive tracts by overeating, which puts too heavy a workload on the digestive system. So moderation is a key factor in regaining health and maintaining it. We have two important rules, the 80/20 quantity rules, for you to keep in mind.

Rule #1:

Eat until your stomach is 80% full, leaving 20% available for digesting.

If you eat until you're 100% full (or even more), this overeating furthers yeast overgrowth. It also slows digestion tremendously. Digestion should occur promptly. If it does not, fermentation occurs, and the yeast happily feed off the sugars produced in the fermentation process. Leaving a little room in the stomach (about 20%) for the digestive enzymes to do their job is essential for efficient digestion and for quickly turning around your body-ecology imbalance.

Rule #2:

80% of the food on your plate should be land and/or ocean vegetables. The remaining 20% can be:

- Animal protein, such as poultry or fish.
- A grain-like seed or a combination of grain-like seeds, such as quinoa with millet.
- A starchy vegetable or combination of starchy vegetables, such as red potatoes and corn.

A typical American meal contains mostly acid-forming foods (such as a big serving of steak or chicken) and not enough alkaline-forming foods, such as non-starchy vegetables. Since candidiasis is an acidic condition, your body needs more alkaline land and ocean vegetables to bring it back into balance.

Again, this also causes a lot of wear and tear on your digestive tract. By following the 80/20 and the food-combining rules, you will never again leave the table feeling over-full and bloated. You won't want to take a nap after a meal, you won't have gas, and you will feel calm and satisfied.

Grains, like wheat and rice, are not on the Body Ecology Diet because fermentation of the natural complex sugars in grain encourages candida overgrowth. *So never, never fill up on grains or starchy vegetables.* Even when you eat the grain-like seeds on The Diet, it's best to limit yourself to one serving and if you're still hungry, have another helping of the alkaline-forming land or ocean vegetables you have prepared.

Vegetable soup	80%
Quinoa	20%
Leftover dinner vegetables	80%
Cream of buckwheat with dulse	20%
Sautéed greens and onions	80%
Poached eggs	20%

Another Breakfast Tip:

Having an *all-alkaline* breakfast is also highly recommended. During the night while we are sleeping, our bodies become more acidic, dehydrated, and more contracted. When we awaken, our first meal of the day should consist of alkaline-forming, high-water-content, expansive foods and drinks. Very sour fruits and their juices (from unsweetened cranberries, pomegranates, and black currents) are ideal because they do not feed the yeast. Another perfect solution is a green smoothie or a super-nutrient "green drink" protein powder. With more nutrients than One A Day vitamin supplements, these now quite popular green drinks are a blend of energizing, powerful whole foods and herbs. Very easy to digest and convenient if you're in a hurry, we believe so much in the value of the green drink that we created two green protein powder blends called Vitality SuperGreen and Potent Proteins. They both contain fermented ingredients to help create a healthy inner ecosystem.

Note: You'll be learning about another possible alkaline-forming breakfast food in Chapter 15: The Magic of Kefir.

∽

FIGURE 6
80%/20% Rule #1

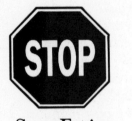

**Stop Eating
When You Are
80% Full**

20%

80%

**Leave 20%
Empty for
Digestion**

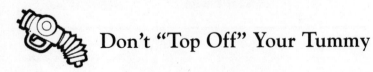

Don't "Top Off" Your Tummy

FIGURE 7
80%/20% Rule #2

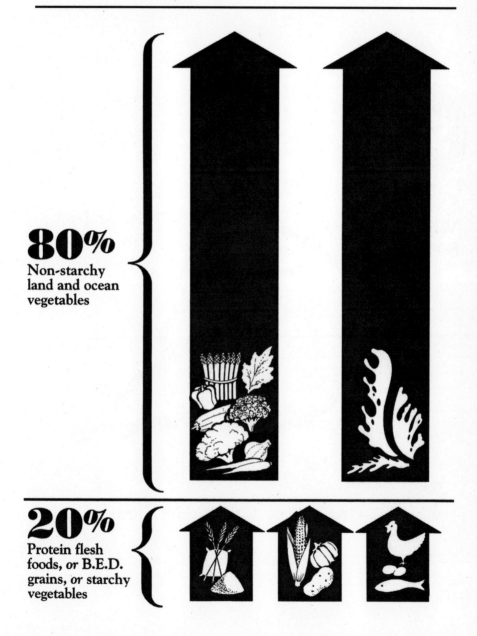

80%
Non-starchy
land and ocean
vegetables

20%
Protein flesh
foods, *or* B.E.D.
grains, *or* starchy
vegetables

Chapter 11

The Principle of Step by Step

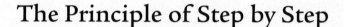

The step-by-step concept intersects with all the other principles, rules, and tips of the Body Ecology Diet; it is one of the most important healing concepts to embrace. Yet it is often overlooked due to its simplicity. It answers the question: how long will it take to heal? In fact, the step-by-step principle is about *time*—taking the time to heal.

Nature acts in a step-by-step, orderly manner, and we cannot violate this order. The life process of birth, maturation, aging, and death illustrates this. A tree must start from a seedling and grow. The seasons of the year have an order that cannot be changed—we cannot go from winter directly to summer without having spring. In spiritual traditions, this is the principle of dawning—dawn occurs little by little in the transition from night to day, and so it goes for all things in nature.

Unfortunately, we often spurn the step-by-step principle, and our health suffers as a result. To illustrate: unwilling to take the time to get over a cold or other cleansings, we take medicine and antibiotics as a "quick cure." In doing this, we halt the body's attempt to eliminate its toxins step by step.

Drugs stop the cleansing process, which the body uses to get rid of illness; drugs drive disease deeper into the body, allowing the potential for an even more serious illness later. But if we permit nature to take its course, cleansing and healing *will* take place, step by step.

We got into trouble when we replaced many home-cooked meals with fast food. Many of us now no longer take the time to learn what cuisine is best for us, to plan menus, shop, and prepare meals. Fast food skips over these steps, resulting in a diet that satisfies our taste and hunger needs, but not our nutritional needs.

The breakdown of our inner body ecology also occurs step by step—in fact, the increments are often so small that we don't even notice them. That's why you can become aware of a yeast overgrowth or a kidney problem, for example, and wonder how it happened all of a sudden. It didn't—it's the result of many assaults to your body ecology over a long period of time. The good news is that healing also takes place in a step-by-step sequence, and all you have to do is start.

How to Heal, Step by Step

You cannot expect instant healing—this too would violate the step-by-step principle. The impurities and toxins you've built up in your system over the years cannot be eliminated all at once—they must be eliminated in an orderly cleansing process. But this doesn't mean it has to be slow. You can choose how quickly you go through the steps of healing. For example, when you first start the Body Ecology Diet, you may have very uncomfortable symptoms of yeast die-off, since you are no longer feeding the yeast. If you absolutely can't stand it, or if you need to feel better for work, you can slow down the cleansing by transitioning into The Diet little by little. Here are some ways you can step more quickly into health:

- Eliminate stress as much as possible.

- Eat according to The Diet—don't cheat!

- Eat foods that especially aid cleansing, such as lemons, limes, raw apple cider vinegar, raw cultured vegetables and young coconut kefir (see Chapters 14 and 15).

- Eliminate medicines that suppress the cleansing process.

- Pay attention to cleansing the colon.

- Rest during periods of cleansing.

- Use probiotics to increase colonies of friendly bacteria.

Even when you take these actions, you will be following the principle of step by step. And in your inner world the colonies of friendly bacteria will be increasing in a step-by-step manner.

Success with The Diet comes step by step. That's why you must be very determined to stick with The Diet until you master it. Develop your willpower, step by step. Advance with The Diet according to your personal pace, the pace that supports you the best. Persevere. When you have a setback—an old symptom or reaction—take only the next step that allows you to get back on track. The beauty of The Diet is that if you do stay with it, you will have success, you *will heal*.

Beginning The Diet is similar to climbing a mountain. When you're at the bottom, at the first step, you can't see the health, happiness, and prosperity that may await you at the top. But as you progress up the mountain, the top reveals itself more and more. As you start The Diet, some things may not be clear, but as you become stronger each day, step by step, your understanding and clarity increase. When you master the principles of The Diet, you'll be at the top of the mountain— vital, knowledgeable, and healthy.

That's why it is important to use your inherent ability to envision yourself in perfect, glowing health, radiating positive energy, feeling strong. By holding this vision, and using The Diet as your guide, you can achieve your goal. If you persist step by step, you will have success.

Just remember how beautiful the world looks from the top of a mountain.

❧

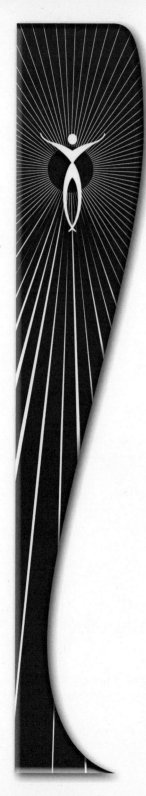

PART III

Description of the Body Ecology Diet

Chapter 12

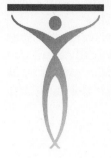

What *Is* the Body Ecology Diet?

Now that you're aware of the basic principles of The Diet, it's time to learn more about what foods are on it and how to combine them properly. You may think it's impossible to incorporate all the principles simultaneously, but as you will see, they all weave automatically and easily into our suggested recipes and menus.

You will be pleasantly surprised by the variety of foods you can eat on The Diet. Some of them may be new to you, so you will have the joy of discovering new tastes and textures. Some (like the ocean vegetables) are different enough that it may take some time to acquire a taste for them. But it will be worth it. Many of the foods have healing qualities, so you will especially want to concentrate on them. And by staying on The Diet, you will feel so much better in such a short time that you will soon be eagerly trying new recipes using its foods.

Because of individual sensitivities, you may find that one or two of the foods on the B.E.D. do not work for you until your immune system is stronger. Don't despair. There are plenty of other foods that you can enjoy.

It's very important that you eat at least three to four meals a day, keeping in mind the 80/20 quantity rules and the principles of The Diet. You may not always feel hungry, but it's necessary to provide your body with these healing foods. This is especially important during periods of cleansing.

The cleansing effect of The Diet often causes weight loss, as stored toxins exit the body's cells. If you are naturally slim, you may even go below your average weight. In time, when your body starts rebuilding, you will regain to your ideal weight, the weight at which your body functions best.

Animal-Protein Foods You Can Eat

Meats, poultry, eggs, and fish are on The Diet. They do not feed fungus. These foods are acid-forming and cause contraction. So to create balance keep in mind the 80/20 rule when serving yourself. Only 20% of your meal should be an animal protein, and 80% should be vegetables. Combining them with raw cultured vegetables is a must. Animal proteins create toxic by-products in the intestines. The microflora in the cultured vegetables turn these toxins back into useful amino acids. They also protect against parasites. If you are willing to eat your animal protein rare or even raw (e.g., salmon or tuna sashimi), you will find it much easier to digest. (If raw, freeze for at least 48 hours to destroy parasites, then defrost.) Buy animal-protein foods that are free from antibiotics and hormones.

At first you need to eat more animal foods than you might like or be accustomed to. A diet too high in animal protein is not healthy, but when you make your initial assault on the yeast, the strengthening quality of animal protein will help balance the expansive nature of Candida Related Complex. Gradually, as the yeast starve and die off, you can increase your grain/vegetable meals and cut down on animal-protein meals. Your blood type offers a clue to how much protein you need. Type A's can transition into a totally vegetarian diet. Type O's will always do best with some animal protein each day, and B's and A/B's will find themselves thriving on moderation—some animal-protein meals and many meals of grain-based entrees.

Remember, fish is the preferred animal-protein food on the B.E.D.; try to have some at least three times a week. Salmon and sardines are especially healthy because of their high content of omega-3 oils, which keep the circulatory system healthy. A well-functioning circulatory system is essential to improving your immunity; the circulatory system carries vital nutrients to all parts of the body and removes waste products.

Eggs

Eggs help strengthen the thyroid, which is often weak in people with candidiasis. Since they are such a concentrated, contracting food, many of us find it best to eat them midday, when the body has plenty of time and energy to digest them. When we wake up in the morning, our bodies are dehydrated and acidic. We need to hydrate and alkalize and create energy to start our day. Eggs can be too heavy and contracting. Still, their strongly contracting nature is grounding and energizing so they can be useful for those with very active mornings.

If you are physically active, they may be the perfect breakfast for you. They wake up the brain and help you focus better. If you are not that active and sit at a desk during the day, it's better to enjoy them between 11 A.M. and 2 P.M. Eggs can be eaten for dinner but are really too contracting and energizing for your last meal of the day. They also take longer to digest than a meal with a grain-like seed, such as quinoa, and your stomach may still be trying to digest them at bedtime. Most people sleep better on an empty stomach, so try to eat your last meal several hours before going to sleep.

One therapeutic way to prepare eggs is to sauté them "over easy" (a soft, runny yolk) in organic, unrefined coconut oil. Then eat only the yolk. The cooked egg white has less nutritional value. Contrary to popular belief, it is the egg yolk that is most healthy.

Softly scrambling one whole egg plus two yolks in butter or ghee is another excellent preparation method.

Eggs are sorely misunderstood these days. Yes, they do have cholesterol, but this is an important fat.[10] The yolk contains lecithin, which aids in fat assimilation. Eggs actively raise the level of HDL, which is the good cholesterol, and they have the most perfect protein components of any food. Today, even though we Americans have cut our egg consumption in half, there has not been a decline in heart disease. If you have been an egg lover and have given them up, you can now enjoy them. Remember to combine them with lots of alkaline vegetables to balance their acidic nature. Raw cultured vegetables (an excellent expansive food) make an ideal balance with the contracting power of eggs. **These enzyme-rich vegetables greatly enhance digestion of protein**. It is also very wise to use a digestive enzyme with HCl and pepsin, which begins digestion in your stomach, and then an enzyme with pancreatin to complete digestion in your small intestine. Many people who test allergic to eggs on allergy tests are simply not digesting them properly. Undigested proteins become a toxin in your digestive tract.

Menu Tip:

Try a land- or ocean-vegetable omelette. Or serve your eggs poached or over easy on a bed of steamed greens. They are delicious scrambled with chopped and sautéed vegetables, such as red onions, summer squashes, scallions, and red bell peppers.

SPECIAL NOTE: With a body-ecology imbalance, animal-protein foods are usually difficult to digest, since hydrochloric acid is often lacking. Here are a few tips to help improve digestion of protein:

- Eat cultured vegetables with every meal! They greatly assist in the digestion of all foods, including proteins.

- Digestive enzymes with hydrochloric acid and pepsin start the digestion of protein in the stomach. Pancreatic enzymes complete this digestion in the small intestine. Digestive enzymes are a must!

- Slowly sip a champagne glass containing one of Body Ecology's probiotic liquids (like InnergyBiotic).

- Sip a glass of water containing two teaspoons of organic apple cider vinegar.

- Cayenne pepper stimulates the secretion of hydrochloric acid. Sprinkle it on your protein foods or cook with it.

A Special Note to Vegetarians:

You can be a *vegan* vegetarian and still conquer candidiasis with the Body Ecology Diet. Just eat the high-protein grain-like seeds (quinoa, millet, buckwheat, and amaranth), along with lots of vegetables, including cultured vegetables and sea vegetables. Practice all seven principles of the B.E.D. You must be especially careful to eat well, not skip meals, and eat a wide variety of foods. Use Celtic sea salt to help make your meals a little more contracting initially, and pay special attention to the popular green drink formulas with their high-protein micro-algae (chlorella, spirulina, dulse, and cereal grasses). Body Ecology has two fermented protein powders: Potent Proteins (with 50% fermented spirulina) and Vitality SuperGreen. Both provide concentrated sources of plant proteins. If you are a lacto-ovo vegetarian, you can eat eggs.

Other Protein Foods (Protein Fats)

Nuts and seeds can be an excellent source of vegetarian protein, but for many people, they can be too difficult to digest. Nevertheless, if you can digest them, you can enjoy them if they are soaked and then eaten raw, dehydrated, or pureed into a paté. Because they are a very concentrated food, eat them in small quantities.

Nuts and seeds are acidic, with the exception of almonds, which are alkaline. Soaking removes an enzyme inhibitor that makes them difficult to digest. Pureeing nuts and seeds after soaking and sprouting makes them much easier to digest.

To soak: Cover nuts or seeds with purified water in a glass or stainless-steel container overnight or for 12 hours. Drain and refrigerate.

To sprout: First soak in a sprouting jar 8–12 hours, then drain. Then turn sprouting jar upside down in your dish drainer for 8 more hours, turning occasionally. The nuts or seeds can then be refrigerated in an airtight container, or use a dehydrator. Sprouting more than one day produces a bitter taste.

Popular seeds eaten on The Diet are flax, chia, sunflower, and pumpkin. Flax and chia seeds have a special mucilage-like compound that helps improve elimination. Each night pour hot water over a tablespoon of the seed of choice and let sit overnight. In the morning, drink everything you see in the cup.

Seeds and nuts fall in the middle, balanced area of the Expansion/Contraction Continuum. Since nuts and seeds are protein fats, they can be eaten with acid fruits, other protein fats (like avocado and milk kefir), and non-starchy, alkaline land and ocean vegetables. Toss a handful into a leafy green salad with an oil and lemon/herb dressing. But remember to chew them well, or better yet, puree them into a paté first.

Grain-like Seeds

The Diet allows four grain-like seeds that are gluten free and do not feed the yeast. You can enjoy millet, quinoa, amaranth, and buckwheat on The Diet. They may not be familiar to you, but they are readily available in health-food stores and some supermarkets. The first three are alkaline-forming. Buckwheat is acid-forming, so cook it with a little bit of good-quality sea salt (which is alkaline) and lots of fresh herbs and vegetables to balance its acidity. All the B.E.D. grain-like seeds are high in protein.

Combine these grains with vegetables (80/20 rule). Eating a grain-like entree for your last meal of the day is ideal, because they digest more quickly than animal foods and you will sleep better at night. Never overconsume these foods; overeating slows down digestion. If they stay in your stomach too long, all grains and grain-like seeds begin fermenting, and this encourages yeast overgrowth.

If your condition is not acute, or once you've become more balanced, you may find that you can tolerate cornmeal, including polenta, corn tortillas, or even small amounts of corn chips. Buy *baked* (no-oil) blue cornmeal chips. Try dipping blue corn chips into a bowl of your favorite cultured vegetables—like you would chips and salsa. They also make a nice crunchy accompaniment to an all-vegetable soup or to vegetable salads.

We are proud of the recipes we've developed for the Body Ecology Diet using the four grain-like seeds. You will notice they usually incorporate land and sea vegetables, making the dishes more nutritious and even easier to digest. Health-food stores also sell flours made from these grains, which allow you even more options as a creative cook. However, the whole seed is much more desirable than the flour. (Flour products are mucus-forming and are harder to digest.) Antifungal herbs, such as turmeric and some curries, make the grain-like seeds even more delicious and more healing.

> *When Mary J. began The Diet, her body ecology was so out of balance that she could not tolerate any cooked grains at all, even the four on the Body Ecology Diet. But by adding cultured foods to her diet, she gradually restored her inner ecosystem and added the four grains, rotating them into her meals one at a time.*

Mary's condition is not uncommon in those with severe cases of candidiasis, especially if the digestive tract is very weak. If you fall into this category, experiment with The Diet's four grains, eliminating the ones that don't work for you. Eat mostly land and ocean vegetables, some animal-protein foods, and **lots of raw cultured vegetables** (more on these below). Focus on cleansing your colon and on introducing plant-based digestive enzymes that are high in amylase. Then slowly introduce the grains, one at a time, to find your tolerance. Eat them in smaller quantities, properly combined with vegetables, and you will do just fine.

An Absolute Must: Soaking

It is always recommended that you soak all grains and grain-like seeds in water for 8 to 24 hours. When the digestive tract is weak and lacking an inner ecosystem, it will not be able to break down the phytic acid found in all grains, beans, nuts, and seeds. Soaking removes this enzyme inhibitor. Do make every effort to eat grain-like-seed meal each day. They add important fiber, help stop cravings for carbs like breads and pastries, and provide valuable nutrients to the microflora struggling to create a new civilization inside your body.

Vegetables

Vegetables are the most perfect foods nature has given us; they are also the most abundant foods on Earth. They are rich in the vitamins and minerals needed to heal the body, and their colors, textures, and shapes add excitement to any meal.

The non-starchy vegetables (see page 62) form excellent combinations with just about every other food. They provide perfect balance to your protein or grain-like-seed meals. They are alkalizing, filling, and give you a sense of well-being and health.

You can eat non-starchy vegetables with organic, unrefined oil; butter; ghee; animal protein; eggs; grains; starchy vegetables (like acorn squash and potatoes); lemons; limes; and protein fats, including almonds and sunflower, caraway, flax, or pumpkin seeds.

Leafy green vegetables, which grow above ground (turnip greens, kale, collards, beet greens), are rich in chlorophyll and help cleanse the blood. They also provide excellent sources of calcium and iron and should be included in every meal. Root vegetables, which grow underground (carrots, onions, daikon, turnips), are more contracting in nature and provide strength and winter warmth.

The *starchy* vegetables, such as red skin new potatoes, water chestnuts, winter squash, artichokes, Jerusalem artichokes, and English peas, can be eaten as entrees and combined only with the four B.E.D. grain-like seeds and the non-starchy vegetables listed above. Red skin potatoes are the only potatoes recommended on The Diet at first; feel free to eat the skins. Sweet corn is only mildly starchy when cooked; if eaten raw, it is a non-starchy vegetable. Fresh or frozen black-eyed peas and lima beans can be eaten if you are able to digest them. They are best digested when combined with non-starchy veggies.

Menu Tip:

A delicious light meal could be baked red skin potatoes topped with ghee, lecithin granules, and herbs, plus a green salad. Potatoes also can be topped with the Body Ecology Diet Gravy (see recipe) or best of all . . . **raw cultured vegetables**.

Ocean Vegetables

Ocean (or sea) vegetables greatly enhance the functioning of the immune system. They are rich in minerals and strengthen the thyroid. The most common ocean vegetables are:

- Agar (AG-GAR)
- Arame (ER-A-MAY)
- Dulse (DULS)
- Hijiki (HE-GEE-KEE)
- Kelp
- Kombu (KOM-BOO)
- Nori (NOR-EE)
- Sea palm
- Wakame (WA-KA-MAY)

You may be most familiar with nori, since sushi bars use nori to wrap and garnish sushi and sushi rolls. Dulse is a chewy snack for many people in the Canadian maritime provinces, where it has been harvested for centuries. Arame is good either cooked or raw. You can add soaked then chopped arame, dulse, or wakame to your salads. Agar is a mild-tasting gelatin used to thicken aspics or puddings; it also helps eliminate constipation. Be sure to cook ocean vegetables with plenty of sweet vegetables, such as onions and carrots, to get a good balance between the sweet and salty tastes.

Besides the recipes we give you, macrobiotic cookbooks have recipes using sea vegetables. Simply adjust them by eliminating the miso and tamari, and replace these ingredients with a little good-quality Celtic sea salt—not too much, since ocean vegetables are naturally salty.

Menu Tip:

You can buy "Sea Seasonings" brand flavorings, such as Dulse with Garlic or Nori with Ginger, to sprinkle on just about everything you cook—soups, main dishes, grains, and salads.

Vegetables Not on the Initial, Therapeutic Version of the Diet

Please don't eat the following vegetables. Here's why:
- Beets (unless cultured), parsnips, sweet potatoes, yams—too high in natural sugars.

- Button mushrooms—too expansive (dried shiitake are fine, however).

- Tomatoes—a fruit, but you may tolerate them occasionally, in season, with a green salad. When cooked, tomatoes become acid-forming. They are not recommended for those with blood types A and B.

- Eggplant and green bell peppers—members of the nightshade family of vegetables, they often irritate the nervous system; people who are highly sensitive or hyperactive should not eat them. Others can eat them in moderation. Green bell peppers are red peppers picked at an early stage. They are very difficult to digest and should not be eaten. Our recipes use only small amounts of red peppers (also nightshades) for flavor and color.

- Russet potatoes—too high in sugar, and feed the yeast.

- Indoor, tray-grown "wheat grass" (really a long sprout)—too sweet, too expansive.

- Mung bean sprouts—typically have mold on them; sunflower and buckwheat sprouts are fine.

Raw vs. Cooked Vegetables

Raw vegetables are an essential source of enzymes, which aid digestion; however, anyone with a weakened digestive tract will find them difficult to digest. (Note: raw cultured vegetables are an exception.) So as you begin The Diet, lightly steamed vegetables may be best for you. Cooked vegetables are slightly warming and more contracting than raw ones, so initially they are better for people whose bodies are in an expanding/weakened condition.

Raw cultured vegetables and raw apple cider vinegar (see below) provide important plant enzymes and greatly enhance digestion. It's important to eat both raw and cooked foods to maintain ideal health. Once you have added fermented foods and beverages to your diet and have restored your inner ecosystem, all foods, both cooked and raw, will be easier to digest.

Try to eat a salad every day using the Body Ecology Diet Dressing, and include at least 1/2 cup of raw cultured vegetables with your meals each day. The raw apple cider vinegar used in all our dressings helps "pre-digest" lettuce, making it easier to assimilate. And both apple cider vinegar and cultured vegetables encourage the growth of friendly bacteria. You'll see a marked improvement in your health once you begin including these items frequently as part of your meals.

Here again, you can use the 80/20 rule: during the colder winter months, or if your digestive tract is weak, eat 80% cooked foods, 20% raw. During the hot summer, and as you become healthier, gravitate toward eating more raw, enzyme-rich vegetables (80% raw and 20% cooked).

A Helpful Hint:

Full-spectrum plant enzymes with protease, amylase, cellulase, and lipase are an excellent digestive aid when eating a vegan (all plant-based) meal. It is wise to also take a pancreatic enzyme with every meal to ensure digestion of proteins, carbohydrates, and fats in your small intestine. Enzymes with hydrochloric acid and pepsin ensure digestion of animal-protein meals (including eggs and dairy) and also nuts and seeds in your *stomach*. But pancreatic enzymes should be taken as well. They ensure digestion of proteins, carbs, and fats once they reach your *small intestine*. High-quality enzymes are available from your health-food store and through Body Ecology. They are a must for everyone, whether healthy or well. They ensure that nutrients are properly assimilated—helping prevent and even correct nutrient deficiencies.

Cooking Tip:

When vegetables are steamed, some of their vitamins and minerals go into the water, so use this water in soups or even drink it to recapture these nutrients.

Fruits

As we've mentioned, the only fruits allowed on The Diet at first are lemons, limes, and berries. Pomegranate, black currant, and cranberry juices are also good for you. They are not sweet enough to feed the yeast. All other fruits are too sweet. After your candida is under control and you start to introduce new foods into your diet, continue eating the so-called sour or acidic fruits—like grapefruit and kiwi. To call them acid fruits is confusing and misleading for many. Indeed they are not acid-forming in your body; they are alkaline-forming.

A VERY IMPORTANT WARNING: Remember the food-combining rule for fruits: eat them alone and on an empty stomach. Lemons and limes, however, are an exception to this rule. You'll find you can use them in salads or squeezed into drinks or on fish and other animal protein with no problem. Watch out for grains and starchy vegetables, though. If you are very sensitive, you may have a problem digesting lemon and lime with grains or grain-like seeds.

You'll find that summer is the best season to eat more fruits. They are cooling and higher in liquids, helping us tolerate the heat.

Green Smoothies and Raw Vegetable Juices

Raw vegetable juices (from certain vegetables) and blended vegetable smoothies provide live enzymes, vitamins, and minerals to help heal your body. These nutrients are in an easily assimilated form and are digested immediately. They help with cleansing and healing long before the nutrients from whole foods begin to work. They are extremely alkaline and expansive—so they are good for balancing acidic, contracting conditions, such as consumption of too much meat. (Visit **www.bodyecology.com** to find delicious Green Smoothie recipes.)

Juicing properly is extremely important. Juices that contain fruits and sweet vegetables (carrots, beets, jicama) feed candida. Juices also lack fiber. Please refer to the chapter on juicing to learn more.

Dairy Products

The milk sugar (lactose) in dairy foods feeds the yeast. The milk sugar (lactose) in dairy foods feeds the yeast. Dairy foods are not only mucus-forming, they also contain the milk protein casein. Casein can leak through a permeable, inflamed gut lining and trigger a negative immune response. Therefore, dairy products are not allowed when you start the B.E.D. Once some of your symptoms disappear, you may be able to tolerate a small amount of *cultured* dairy foods (kefir and yogurt). Yogurt and kefir have very little milk sugar and are usually safe if you are lactose intolerant. Because their protein is pre-digested, they stay in your stomach for a shorter time. If you eat them, enrich your kefir or yogurt with other probiotics such as acidophilus and bifidus (various strains). Combine them with raw and lightly steamed vegetables or cultured vegetables. Digestive enzymes that support digestion of milk products in both the stomach and the small intestine are a must. To learn why we prefer kefir to yogurt, see page 134.

Herbs

Most herbs are welcome on The Diet. If you can get organically grown herbs, so much the better. You can season your dishes with basil, bay leaves, cayenne, chives, coriander, cumin, curry, dill, garlic powder, ginger, Italian and Mexican seasonings, mustard powder, marjoram, oregano, black pepper, poppy seeds, rosemary, sage, tarragon, and thyme.

Herbs that are particularly healing include cayenne, curry, ginger, and garlic.

Here are some brand-name herb products we recommend:

- "Sea Seasonings" (flavors: Dulse, Dulse with Garlic, Nori with Ginger, Kelp with Cayenne)
- "Herbamare" (blend of herbs and sea salt)
- "Trocomare" (sea salt, blend of herbs, and cayenne pepper)

Experiment with your favorite herbs and tastes as you try the recipes on The Diet. You can have a new taste experience just about every day as you vary what you cook and how you cook it.

Sea Salt

Refined table salt has gotten a justly deserved bad reputation during these times of concern about hypertension and heart disease. But if a mineral-rich sea salt is used correctly, it enhances the healing value of foods, besides enhancing their flavor.

The Diet uses mineral-rich sea salts medicinally, to help restore the body's balance. Since candidiasis is a condition of too much expansion and acidity, small amounts of mineral-rich sea salt help contract and alkalize the body, bringing it into balance. That's why some of the more contracting foods, such as poultry, eggs, and even meat (containing salts), are desirable when you first start The Diet.

Sea salt should always be added to the cooking water of grains and grain-like seeds to make them less acid-forming. You can use a small amount of salt (just enough to heighten the natural flavors) in the final 10 to 15 minutes of cooking a soup or vegetables. When cooked for 10 minutes or more, salt chelates, blending with other foods, and does not cause such a "salty" reaction in our bodies.

We recommend high-quality sea salts in our Body Ecology kitchens. Our favorites are from Selina Naturally (**www.selinanaturally.com**). Celtic sea salt is great for cooking, while their Hawaiian sea salt is excellent to sprinkle over your food at the table. Selina Naturally also sells a special salt grinder for table use, one with non-metallic parts that won't interact with the salt. These can also be found in most cookware stores.

Men and women have different needs for salt; men need a little more of sea salt's contracting quality. Women should cut way back on salt and continue to do so from the time of ovulation until they complete their period (monthly cleansing) so their bodies will easily "open up," relax, and expand ever so slightly to release the uterine lining. When a woman's body becomes too contracted from too much sea salt, she will have extreme cravings for sugary, sweet foods as her body attempts to balance itself so the lining of the uterus can be shed. If she eats too much salt during her period, she may not have a complete cleansing. After the lining is shed, a woman can increase her use of sea salt and contracting foods a bit (which will help bring on a smooth ovulation). She should still balance the contracting foods with some expanding foods, of course. The more contracting foods are best to eat close to the time of ovulation. Doing so helps the ovary contract and the tiny egg "pop out."

Non-alcoholic Flavorings

Non-alcoholic liquid flavorings can be used on the Body Ecology Diet, especially in dessert recipes. Look for glycerine-based natural extracts such as almond, vanilla, banana, pineapple, and even coffee. Some have a vegetable oil (soybean) base, and some have a vegetable/glycerine oil base. The 100% glycerine-based flavorings are the ones you want. You might find that you are sensitive to one flavoring and not another, but usually these should work for you. The extracts are made by squeezing the essential oils from foods and putting them with these bases. These oils have no sugar; therefore, they don't feed the yeast. That's why you can safely use fruit flavors such as pineapple or banana (unless you are somehow sensitive to the carrier oil).

Most health-food stores stock these flavorings or can order them for you.

Fermented Foods

The Body Ecology Diet is a gluten-free, sugar-free, probiotic-rich diet. We encourage you to eat plenty of the most healing of foods . . . fermented foods. The real "stars" of The Diet are a variety of fermented or *cultured* vegetables and a magical fermented drink called young coconut kefir. Fermenting the meat of the young coconut gives us another fermented food called coconut kefir "cheese." Body Ecology also has fermented protein powders and probiotic liquids. Thankfully, fermented foods are gaining much-deserved attention and a worldwide reputation for being magical healing foods.

The Body Ecology–approved cultured foods fight yeast and other unhealthy pathogens in your intestines. Besides providing your body with beneficial microflora (bifidus, acidophilus, plantarum, bulgaricus, and beneficial yeast), these cultured foods will be an important factor in recolonizing your inner ecosystem.

Apple cider vinegar is another fermented food that is also on The Diet. Look for unfiltered vinegar packaged in light-proof or dark opaque containers. This prevents photo-oxidation and protects the integrity of the product. Look for products that tell you on the label that they are raw, unpasteurized, and contain the "mother" of the vinegar.

Avoid such fermented foods as salted and pasteurized sauerkraut. This sauerkraut is nothing like the microflora-rich, cultured vegetables on The Diet. Amasake, a fermented rice drink, has too much sugar. Kombucha tea and Rejuvelac contain wild yeast that produce dangerous toxins. Milk kefir, a fermented food, is discussed in detail in a later chapter.

Rich in potassium and alkaline-forming, apple cider vinegar is an "antidote" when you've had too much salt or sugar. It's delicious in the Body Ecology Diet Salad Dressing, and you can use it to substitute for other vinegars in various recipes (even homemade mayonnaise). You can have mustard if it is made with raw apple cider vinegar (see Shopping List in Appendix A for brand names).

Cultured vegetables are ones that have been cut or shredded and left in an airtight sanitary environment for several days or longer at room temperature. This lets the lactobacilli and enzymes that are naturally present on the vegetables proliferate, creating an enzyme-rich, mineral-rich super food that aids digestion, eliminates toxins, and restores or maintains a healthy inner ecosystem. **Cultured vegetables are wonderful for controlling sugar cravings**.

You can make your own cultured vegetables or buy them in health-food stores. We recommend you have at least 1/2 cup a day as you begin The Diet, especially with your protein or grain meals. We cannot emphasize enough the value of these precious foods.

Fermenting foods may seem time-consuming, but they are simple to prepare and well worth the effort. They are also a very economical way to reestablish your inner ecosystem, since they cost far less than expensive probiotics.[12]

If you have a few friends or family members on The Diet, spend a Sunday afternoon together making cultured vegetables and young coconut kefir. Breaking up the work and talking makes the time pass quickly (see Chapters 14 and 15 for more on these foods).

A SPECIAL WORD OF CAUTION: Cultured veggies are loaded with beneficial bacteria that are intensely interested in cleaning up their new environment . . . your intestines. There, in their brave new world, they will do everything in their power to fulfill their mission . . . co-creating with you to craft a healthy, beautiful body. They go to work immediately softening hardened fecal material, attacking toxins, combating parasites, and balancing the acidity/alkalinity of both intestines. While this is actually an excellent arrangement for you, it often creates gas and bloating. The solution? Rinse out the toxic material with daily home enemas or schedule yourself for a series of colonics. Keep eating cultured foods, and once this initial stage of cleansing passes, you'll look and feel great. Trust the cleansing principle. Trust the microflora that protect and provide for you.

Water

Pure, high-quality drinking water is critical to recovering your health. Your system needs at least six to eight 8-ounce glasses each day. Try to drink half of these by mid-morning, to make up for the fluids your body missed during the night. If drinking water is not easy for you because you don't like it, flavor it. Adding stevia and a slice of lemon to your drinking water works well.

If you don't drink fluids during the day because you're too busy and forget, wear a timer that signals you to take a few sips from a nearby container. Most people underestimate the amount of water they drink in a day, so count your glasses.

It's especially important to consume more water if you are taking one of the popular fiber products that help improve elimination, like a flaxseed fiber blend. (We recommend 4Fiber by Genesis Today.) Psyllium (not recommended) can be especially binding and can cause constipation without adequate water.

Do you often find yourself full of energy just around bedtime, so you stay up too late and then feel exhausted the next morning? This condition can be a sign of simply not drinking enough water during the day. We sleep poorly when we are dehydrated.

It's essential to drink pure, good-quality water. Chlorine and fluoride destroy the friendly bacteria in your digestive tract. Only drink filtered water. Sparkling mineral water is acceptable on The Diet. (Gerolsteiner and Apollinaris are our favorites.)

Cravings for sugar are often a sign of dehydration. Drink a couple of glasses of water before you give in to that craving and you probably won't want those sweets after all.

The Herb Stevia

About 16 years ago when I (Donna) set off on a quest to find a healthy sweetener that would not spike blood sugar or feed candida, I learned of stevia.

The stevia plant, a small shrub and member of the chrysanthemum family (closely related to chamomile and tarragon), is 200 to 300 times sweeter than sugar. It has been used for centuries by the Guarani Indians of South America, where it grows naturally. Stevia has a long history of safe and therapeutic use as an herbal sweetener and as an antifungal, anti-inflammatory, and antibiotic agent.

At that time, stevia was all but unknown here in the US. Fortunately, however, Jim May (who founded Wisdom Natural Brands) had begun to import stevia here as an unrefined green herb. The leaves were sold crushed in bulk form, were made into a green concentrate, or were crushed and used in tea bags to sweeten tea formulas. Because of the strong licorice-like taste, I knew that stevia, in this form, would never replace sugar.

Searching further (and with a touch of serendipity), I came across the *white extract powder* from China and Japan.

Forty years ago the Japanese discovered how to extract the two sweet elements in stevia, rebaudioside A and stevioside, from the *unrefined green leaf,* creating the safest, most natural calorie-free sweetener. Up until recently Japan consumed more stevia than any other country, using it as a food additive in soft drinks, juices, chewing gum, pickles, frozen desserts, bean and fish paste products, and low-calorie foods.

Because I had a chapter in the first edition of *The Body Ecology Diet* book devoted to the use of stevia, I secured an extremely high-quality stevia/rebaudioside *extract powder*, but as soon as it arrived in the US, the FDA put a ban on importing stevia in any form.

Since I already had it and knew that people would benefit from this amazing natural sweetener, I decided to take the risk and introduce stevia/rebaudioside extract to the country. I began to educate people about its history and safety; wrote *The Stevia Cookbook*; and created a very successful grassroots movement, turning tens of thousands of people on to stevia with the help of proponents Doctors Robert Atkins, Andrew Weil, and Julian Whitaker.

When the FDA lifted the ban, stevia immediately appeared on the shelves in the supplement section of health-food stores labeled as a dietary supplement . . . but not as a sweetener. It took until December 2008, with a petition by Coca-Cola, for the FDA to recognize rebaudioside A (the sweeter component of stevia) as a safe general-purpose sweetener.

All forms of stevia have been tested extensively in human and animal studies around the world with no negative side effects.

When you read about the medicinal attributes of stevia such as helping balance blood sugar by balancing the pancreas, or that stevia helps regulate the digestive tract to produce a healthy stool, and that it greatly increases energy, this is referring to the *unrefined green herb*. The white powder extract would not have these properties.

In Japan, South Korea, Argentina, Brazil, China, and other countries, both stevia and its extract have been recommended for diabetics. Now with the FDA approving stevia here in the US, many other countries are following suit. The good news is that after 16 years of winning the hearts of millions here in the US, stevia/rebaudioside as a sweetener is here to stay . . . a victory worth celebrating. As stevia continues to win the hearts of more Americans, aspartame and other artificial sweeteners are quickly vanishing from our diet.

All forms of stevia significantly reduce the potential for cavities.[13]

All forms of stevia inhibit sugar cravings, which can lure you off The Diet.

Stevia is wonderful in teas, in Body Ecology's probiotic beverages, and as a sweetener in quinoa flakes cooked into a cereal for breakfast. It is especially delicious with the flavor of fruit and with dairy foods. However, it is not as versatile for baking. For baking we recommend Lakanto from Japan (**www.bodyecology.com**).

Getting just the right amount of sweetness can be tricky. After a couple of years I realized that working with the white powder was difficult for most people, so I created the first white stevia liquid concentrate from the white *extract*. Body Ecology's Liquid Stevia Concentrate™ uses only the finest-quality rebaudioside and stevia extracts. It is then filtered to remove the licorice-like aftertaste. It is easy to use and is quite delicious, with the perfect amount of sweetness. Naturally we love it when many people tell us that ours is the most delicious-tasting stevia on the market today.

NOTE: I (Donna) have created more than 100 stevia recipes for *The Stevia Cookbook*, but many are not recommended for someone on the first (or healing) stage of the Body Ecology Diet. (French Chocolate Ice Cream or Cheesecake would be an example.) They also use the white extract powder. See much more on stevia in Part VII: Special Foods, Recipes & Menu Suggestions. Please also visit our stevia website at: **Stevia.net**.

Teas

Several teas are especially healing and antifungal: mathake, echinacea, and pau d'arco (also known as Brazilian bark or Taheebo). You can have as much of these as you want! Also healing are Burdock root and dandelion-root teas and Yogi Digest-Ease tea. Avoid fruit teas and teas with citric acid.

Green tea and ginger tea enhance digestion. Body Ecology's tea concentrates with stevia are delicious and very convenient. At restaurants, when traveling, or at home and work, simply add 30–40 drops of our tea concentrate to hot or cold water for caffeine-free, sugar-free instant tea.

Homemade Ginger Tea

Boil several slices of ginger root in one quart of water for about 15–20 minutes. Add stevia to taste, and lemon juice if you desire. Let the tea sit for a half hour or more. You can make it stronger or weaker depending on your taste.

Unrefined Organic Seed Oils

Organic, unrefined seed oils are great culinary oils and add wonderful flavors and medicinal value to your meals. Unrefined seed oils along with extra-virgin olive oil, coconut oil, butter, and ghee, are definitely on The Diet. In fact, these fats and oils when used together create a special synergy. Each fat or oil has a different fatty-acid profile. The combination of all these fatty acids when taken together is what makes them so healing.

The unrefined seed oils allowed on The Diet are safflower, sunflower, pumpkin seed, hemp seed, evening primrose, borage, and flax.

All the organic, unrefined seed oils on the B.E.D. are rich in omega-6 fatty acids. Most of us obtain ample amounts of omega-6, but it is in the omega-3s that we are often seriously deficient in. Both omega-6 and omega-3 essential fatty acids must be obtained from our food since they are not made by our bodies. Besides being good sources of energy, these fatty acids play a key role in how oxygen is carried throughout our bodies. Found in high concentrations in the brain, they are important for normal brain function, the transmission of nerve impulses, and the regulation of our hormones. Fish oils are excellent sources of omega-3s, so they should also be included in your diet to help create balance to the seed oils. Flax seed oil is our richest vegetarian source of omega-3s from the plant kingdom. Research now shows that by adding unrefined essential fatty acid (EFA) oils to a healthy diet such as the Body Ecology Diet, normal weight can be restored in obese people. In order for this to work, though, all refined oils and margarine must be removed from the diet.[15] Other benefits showing up in the latest research on using these oils with a diet like ours are: a stronger immune system; an increase in energy; normal blood cholesterol levels; healthier eyes; soft, pliable skin; and relief from pain and arthritis. These oils are being used in alternative medical clinics and spas around the world to fight depression, emotional disorders, ADHD, autism, and even schizophrenia.

One of our favorite oils is unrefined pumpkin seed oil. It is delicious, is very nutritious, and even has certain medicinal properties. It has been traditionally used to nourish and heal the digestive tract, fight parasites, improve circulation, and help heal prostate disorders. It also helps nourish the ovaries and prevent dental decay. Pretty amazing for a delicious-tasting oil, isn't it?

Therapeutically, one to two tablespoons of unrefined EFA oils should be taken at least once a day. To protect the heat-sensitive omega-3s, do not cook with them. They can be used in salad dressings and dribbled over your vegetables and grain-like seeds. Coconut oil, butter, and ghee are best for sautéing. (Olive oil can also be used for cooking if you use a low temperature.) Use them in salad dressings, or sprinkle them generously on your fish or chicken. Dribble them onto grains, baked potatoes, leafy greens, ocean and cultured veggies, or a B.E.D. soup once it has cooled down enough to eat. Buy organic, unrefined oils in dark light-proof bottles.

Coconut Oil, Butter, Ghee

Cook with organic, unrefined coconut oil. Contrary to the misinformation put out by the hydrogenated-soy-oil industries, coconut oil is actually a beneficial fat. It contains lauric acid, an important fatty acid (found abundantly in mother's milk) that has an antiviral effect in the body. Coconut oil is excellent for the thyroid and does not raise cholesterol when consumed in a diet that contains essential fatty acids (flax oil, etc.). Coconut oil is naturally stable and therefore excellent for sautéing. Also important to note for anyone suffering from candida: coconut oil is a rich source of caprylic acid, a potent antifungal.

You can also sauté with butter or ghee. Ghee is clarified butter, the *oil* of butter with the milk solids removed. (It's the milk solids in regular butter that contain those harmful hormones and antibiotics.) Ghee is less mucus-forming than butter and contains no lactose (milk sugar), so it is ideal for an anti-candida diet. Cooking with a mixture of half unrefined coconut oil and half ghee produces a delicious flavor. Ghee keeps longer than butter and does not require refrigeration.

You can make your own ghee. Here's how: Melt two to four 1/4-pound sticks of butter in a saucepan over medium/low heat. It will start bubbling, and you will see the white milk solids gather on the surface. Then these solids start to clear away from the surface. Allow this clearing to continue for a couple of minutes (too long and the ghee will burn). Remove pan from heat, and let it cool. The solids will sink to the bottom, and you can strain the clear yellow liquid into a jar. It keeps fine at room temperature or in the refrigerator.

The best butter to eat is *raw, organic* butter. Unfortunately, its sale is now prohibited in most of the 50 states. Raw butter is better because it contains the enzyme lipase, which helps digest the fat in the butter. It is lighter in color and has a delicious flavor. Today, if you want the best butter possible, you'll have to make it yourself. And that is easier to do than you might think. Body Ecology's Culture Starter can be used to make *cultured* butter. The hardy microflora in the starter pre-digest the butter fat. Simply add our starter to organic cream (raw, if possible) and let it sit at room temperature for 24 hours. Then chill it, and beat it with an electric whisk, pouring off any liquid that forms. (This liquid is cultured buttermilk.) Suddenly you'll have delicious *cultured butter*.

Residents of some states can purchase raw cream in their health-food stores and can make butter that is both *raw* and *cultured*. Those living in states that prohibit the retail sale of raw dairy products can often buy them directly from the farmer. (Visit **www.realmilk.com** for more info.)

Avoid margarine. The hydrogenation process used in manufacturing margarine creates trans-fatty acids that are harmful to your health.

Fat Intolerance

Until your inner ecosystem is restored, your liver improves, and your digestive tract is teeming with fat-digesting friendly bacteria, you may not be able to tolerate oils, butter, or fats at all and will have to avoid them completely. This is very common with a body-ecology imbalance because of the toxic, congested condition of the liver and gallbladder. Symptoms of fat intolerance are: pains in the neck and shoulders; spasms in the large and small intestines; feeling tired just after eating; bloating, indigestion, belching, flatulence, and/or nausea; right upper abdominal discomfort; and hard stools. Fat intolerance can be confirmed by a simple urine test or by simply eliminating fats from your diet for a week and noting any improvement in your digestion and your energy.

As you continue on The Diet and keep eating lots of fermented foods and drinks, you'll find that fats and oils are easier to digest. Digestive enzymes that help digest fat (like Body Ecology's Assist SI) should be taken with each meal.

A small amount of organic, unrefined coconut oil used for sautéing (as for onions when making a pot of soup) shouldn't cause you any discomfort; salad dressings or butter on your potato may. Fortunately, we have solved this problem for you. Take a look at the recipe section in Part VII to learn how to make no-oil salad dressings. The oil has been replaced with water and xanthan gum—a natural, flavorless thickener tolerated by everyone and available at health-food stores.

Good news: The microflora in fermented foods produce B vitamins. B-3, B-6, and B-12 play a critical role in the assimilation of fats. Once your inner ecosystem is established with lots of vitamin B–producing friendly bacteria, you'll find it easier to digest fats.

Heart Healthy

While the Body Ecology Diet is enjoying a worldwide reputation as the premier diet for treating candidiasis and immune disorders, it is certainly an excellent eating program for everyone. People with heart conditions and cholesterol problems find The Diet is great for them as well. If you or someone you love has high cholesterol, eat plenty of the following:

- Fermented foods and liquids with friendly bacteria and beneficial yeast—daikon (a large white Chinese radish) helps dissolve bad fats

- Green smoothies and raw vegetables in large salads

- Lemons, berries, and the juices of sour fruits like pomegranate

- Garlic and ginger

- Fresh fish (salmon, halibut, and white fish)

- The B.E.D. organic, unrefined oils (coconut, olive, and fish oils are especially valuable)

- Lecithin

Reminder: Enjoy adequate, consistent amounts of the very highest-quality coconut oil, butter, ghee, and unrefined vegetable oils with proteins; grain-like seeds; and starchy, non-starchy, and ocean vegetables. But be cautious when eating too much animal protein. Excessive amounts of fats—even the ones on The Diet—delay the secretion of gastric juices that digest animal proteins. This means those all-American tuna, egg, and chicken salads with a lot of mayo are out. (See recipe section for no-oil dressings you can use if desired.) **Digestion of fats is greatly enhanced when they are eaten with cultured vegetables, daikon, leafy green salads, apple cider vinegar, and lemon juice**.

Extra-virgin, raw olive oil has valuable heart-protective qualities including vitamin E and important antioxidants, but only trace amounts of essential fatty acids. Most everyone can enjoy this excellent oil right from the beginning. However, if you are very sensitive to fats, you may have to wait a few weeks until you have introduced fermented foods into your diet.

Olive oil is from a fruit (not a seed), and fermented olives can contain mold.

A Summary of the Foods to Avoid on the Body Ecology Diet

- Sugars—including honey, molasses, corn syrup, dextrose, brown rice syrup, barley malt, etc.—feed the yeast.

- Alcohol—is dehydrating and acidic and creates more yeast.

- Breads, flour products, and grains (except those discussed in this chapter)—contain gluten, a protein that causes an autoimmune reaction in someone with yeast infections, and their natural sugars feed the yeast.

- Citric acid found in many foods and teas (read labels).

- Legumes, beans, and peanuts—too difficult to digest, and they cause fermentation and sugars; peanuts attract fungus during processing.

- Mushrooms—encourage allergic reactions (dried shiitake is okay).

- Nut butter and nut milk (including almond milk)—both are too acid-forming and often contain sugar. Nut butters are difficult to digest.

- Oils (other than those discussed in this chapter)—e.g., refined, bleached deodorized canola, soybean, peanut, and toasted sesame.

- Yeast—baker's and brewer's—causes allergic reactions.

Words of Encouragement

You may think there are more "do's and don'ts" on this diet than you can possibly handle—but don't worry! After a little practice, eating according to The Diet will become second nature to you. Just remember that The Diet absolutely works, and it takes different amounts of time for different people to feel better.

Free a free copy of Body Ecology's
Quick Start Guide, go to:
www.BodyEcology.com

❧

Notes

[10] Jennings-Sauer, 1988.

[11] Although beets are not normally on the B.E.D., they are okay in this instance, because the friendly bacteria in the cultured vegetables devour the sugar in the beets and, therefore, the sugar is no longer available to feed the yeast.

[12] The money spent on probiotics, however, is well worth it, especially in your first year of healing. Before they start The Diet, many people spend a lot of money on various avenues of healing. Instead, spend your money on high-quality foods recommended by The Diet, and on cultured vegetables and high-quality probiotics.

[13] Dr. Kleber, Dental Science Research Group, Purdue University.

[14] Roberts, 1990.

[15] We've included a recipe for a B.E.D. mayonnaise, but please remember that mayonnaise is not a *healing food* and should be eaten sparingly—reserved only for special occasions.

Chapter 13

Juicing

Machines that grind fresh raw fruits and vegetables into juices seem to be everywhere these days: in the stores, on television, and featured in books touting their many benefits. It's a great sign that people want to include healthier foods in their diets and reap the rewards of the vitamins, minerals, and enzymes in fresh produce. But juicing is not the panacea it's often portrayed to be, and for people with body-ecology imbalances, it may even aggravate their symptoms especially if they start juicing too soon.

Is Juicing Good for You?

Yes and no. Juices, if made properly, can play a significant role in healing (especially of the liver—see Chapter 21). The key is learning how to prepare them properly and use the right ingredients.

Benefits of Juicing

•   Juices can balance an overly contracted condition. Because of their high water content, they are the most expansive form of fruits and vegetables. You can use them medicinally to correct contracted conditions, including constipation, headaches brought on by too much salt, and the irritability and moodiness some women experience before their periods. A stressful lifestyle causes contraction; so does airplane travel. Freshly prepared juices can bring your body right back into balance.

•   The alkaline-forming nature of juices, if made properly, can balance an acidic condition and aid in cleansing. Regular consumption of juices strengthens all bodily functions by keeping the organs, glands, and cells clean and free of the toxins that create an acidic condition. Again, juices, with their high water content, catalyze cleansing.

•   Juices are easily digested and nutrient-rich. Raw juices are as rich in the same nutrients, oxygen, water, and enzymes as the whole fruits and vegetables from which they're made. Thus, these important nutrients become much more readily available, an enormous benefit for people with nutrient deficiencies.

•   Juices give the digestive tract a much-needed rest. Within minutes of being consumed, they send a quick source of fuel into the bloodstream, allowing the digestive organs to take a break. The tremendous amount of energy that would be spent on digestion can then be used for cleansing and rebuilding the body.

Then Why Not Juice?

It can be costly. To do it right, you need to purchase an expensive piece of equipment ($100 to $300 or more). You'll also be buying enormous quantities of fresh vegetables (fruit juices, with a few exceptions, are not on The Diet). Preparing the vegetables—washing and feeding them into the juicer—takes time. And cleaning the machine can be a nuisance.

Juices separate out the fiber; without fiber, they are digested quickly, and this can be a problem. (See Rule #2 on the next page.)

Equally important is the fact that once juiced some vegetables and most fruits have a high concentration of natural sugars and therefore feed yeast and opportunistic organisms. They do not alkalize. In fact, they make your body more acidic instead and your yeast infection becomes worse.

Because they assimilate so quickly, juices do not combine well with any other food. If they are eaten with protein or starches, which take much longer to digest, they will cause digestive problems including fermentation and gas. How can you overcome these negatives and make juicing work for you?

Timing Is Everything

There are SIX important rules to remember:

Rule #1:

Don't juice until your yeast problem is completely under control.

Wait until you have implanted significant colonies of friendly bacteria into your digestive tract. You should also see other signs that your body ecology is back in balance—for example, all symptoms of yeast overgrowth should be gone. For most people, this takes at least three months. Remember, you don't want to feed the yeast any form of sugar. When you're ready to try juices, introduce them cautiously, as you would any other new food, and watch for signs that your body might not be ready yet.

Rule #2:

Add something to slow down the absorption of the raw vegetables.

1) Fiber, including chia seeds and flax fiber; 2) unrefined, organic oils, including coconut oil and flax seed oil blends;

3) protein powders, including Potent Proteins and Vitality SuperGreen from Body Ecology; 4) a protein fat such as a splash of milk kefir, avocado, soaked and finely ground nuts or seeds, the fermented coconut meat that we call "coconut kefir cheese," or a small spoonful of nut butter, if you digest it. Colostrum powder might work for you as well. Add only those ingredients that work best for your unique body.

Rule # 3:

Avoid vegetables from the cruciferous family, like kale and cabbage.

These vegetables will suppress your thyroid and cool your body too much. It is difficult to rid your body of yeast when the temperature is too low. And when your thyroid is underactive you lose the energy you need to heal.

Rule #4:

Avoid sweet vegetables (such as beets, carrots, and jicama) and most fruits.

Rule #5:

Create juices where all the ingredients digest well together.

(See Rule #2 above for suggestions.)

Rule #6:

Drink juice only on an empty stomach.

Drink juice as your first meal of the day. Wait at least 45 minutes before eating anything else.

Why are these rules necessary? Read on.

Vegetable Juices

To make most vegetable juices more palatable, carrots or another sweet vegetable are usually added. And concentrated carrot juice yields a very strong sugar. So juice blends that have a sweet base of carrot, beet, jicama, and/or fennel must follow the food-combining rule for sugar, which is to eat it alone on an empty stomach at least one half hour before any other solid food. And if your yeast overgrowth is not under control, the sugar will feed it, causing a flare-up of symptoms, and you could lose the ground you've gained.

Juices made only with greens and noncruciferous vegetables (celery, romaine lettuce, zucchini) and non-starchy, low-sugar, high-water-content vegetables such as cucumbers do not have to follow this special food-combining rule. However, juices assimilate so rapidly, it is still always best to "chew them" alone, wait the half hour, and then eat your other foods.

"Chewing" your juice means to hold it in your mouth, allowing the digestion process to begin by mixing it with saliva. Savoring your vegetable juices in this way makes a huge difference. Adding a bit of flax fiber is also wise so that the juice assimilates more slowly.

Fruit Juices

Like fresh fruit, fruit juices are rich in natural sugars and are not on the Body Ecology Diet, with the exception of lemons; limes; black currants; cranberries; and (this one will surprise you) Granny Smith apples, which have much less sweetness than juiced carrots and make a better base for the raw juiced vegetables. Although it is a fruit, this sour green apple is compatible with all vegetable juices. To ensure that it does not cause a problem with the yeast, we also combine it with freshly squeezed lemon juice. The recipe at the end of this chapter is an excellent example of a juice blend that is not only surprisingly tasty, but healing as well.

You can have these juices on an empty stomach at least one half hour before eating other foods.

A glass of unsweetened cranberry juice or black currant juice diluted with water and sweetened with stevia is excellent for strengthening the bladder and alleviating urinary tract infections. Recent research shows that compounds in cranberry juice prevent pathogenic (unfriendly) bacteria from adhering to the bladder walls. Black currant juice is excellent for the adrenals (noni and pomegranate juice are now available as well).

Lemon juice and lime juice, or a combination of the two, are natural antiseptics and cleanse the digestive tract. The very sour fruit juices help stimulate the peristaltic action of the colon and promote morning bowel movements. Once you begin introducing new foods, you can also try grapefruit juice from the more sour varieties of the fruit.

More Tips on How to Make Juicing Work for You

Be creative! Substitute lemon juice and/or a small amount of sour green apple juice for sweet vegetables (carrots, beets, fennel). Combine a high concentration of celery, plus a smaller amount of cucumber, or romaine lettuce and parsley. As mentioned earlier, stay away from cabbage, kale, and collards because in their raw form they suppress the thyroid.

When necessary, dilute some of the sweetness in your juice by adding water, either spring or filtered, and/or lemon juice.

Wheat grass juice is rich in sugar and is too expansive. It often causes nausea or dizziness. However, it's great after an enema or colonic.

Try to juice only what you will drink right away; do not make extra. If it sits around, even in the refrigerator, it becomes more sugary. If you must juice for several meals at one time, keep the green apple juice in a separate container from the other juices. Mix together just before drinking.

Add herbs, such as parsley, cilantro, basil, mint, and even watercress. You don't need a lot of these, but their high concentration of chlorophyll will help cleanse your blood and cells and add a lot of flavor.

Juices can also taste savory, especially if you add herbs like chives and sea veggies. Sea Seasonings brand Dulse with Garlic or Kelp with Cayenne are both great additions to enhance the taste and nutrients in your vegetable juice. When concerned about the sweetness of a juice, simply add a teaspoon to a tablespoon of apple cider vinegar to achieve balance. Use a couple of drops of stevia liquid concentrate to sweeten. A dash of sea salt helps create more balance.

Add friendly bacteria to your juice. Acidophilus, bifidus, and the lactobacillus and good yeast in kefir are great components of a healthy juice. Milk kefir combines well with acid fruits and raw vegetables. Our probiotic liquids and young coconut kefir always enhance any juice recipe.

The Bottom Line

Juice fasting for a day can be very beneficial. Try it on a day when you can stay at home and rest. Drink a lot of juice often so you don't get weak. Colon cleansing—colonics or enemas—is important during this time. Because of the cleansing effect of the juices, the colon wants to release more stagnant material than normal peristaltic movement will allow. If you want to fast longer, consult with a health-care professional who's an expert on fasting.

Juicing can be very beneficial as long as you follow the rules. The investment of your time and money now will pay off in years of better health for you and savings in health-care costs later in life.

The following juice recipe is an ideal mixture of good health and good taste. Most juices with this much chlorophyll are unpalatable, but ours, when mixed with a little Granny Smith apple juice, is delicious. Drinking the juices immediately after juicing is ideal, but because of the time and effort it takes to clean and juice vegetables, most of us find this very inconvenient. We have found that as long as you keep the green mixture separate from the apple juice, this green juice recipe will last for two to three days.

Celery—50%

Zucchini—30%

Romaine lettuce—10%

Parsley—5%

Granny Smith apple—5% (juiced separately and added)

Ground flax fiber

Ginger to taste (optional)

Mix together green veggie mixture with green apple juice plus add the juice of half a lemon. Splash in a dash of sea salt and/or finely ground dulse. Enjoy!

Reminder:

Juicing at the beginning of The Diet and juicing improperly can set you back seriously. Once your body ecology is restored, you may try introducing fresh vegetable juices very cautiously—always on an empty stomach first thing in the morning. Wait half an hour before eating other food.

Vitality SuperGreen, our alkalizing green food blended with nutrients to nourish your intestines, is an excellent drink for you even as you begin The Diet. It is delicious when added to a juice of all green vegetables. Taken alone with water, it can be a quick energy-boosting meal. In the morning for breakfast, it is a convenient way to start the day; taken in the late afternoon, it's a quick pick-me-up and revitalizer.[16] Potent Proteins, which contains 50% fermented spirulina and 50% fermented B.E.D. grain-like seeds, can be used in the same way.

Green Smoothies Are a Better Choice Than Juicing

Both blended vegetable *smoothies* and vegetable *juices* will provide you with a raw food meal that is loaded with nutrients and enzymes. We humans lack the enzyme to digest the cellulose fiber in raw vegetables. Blending veggies makes them much easier to digest. (Cooking does this, too.)

By now we all know that fiber is good for us. Remember when you remove the fiber, vegetable juice metabolizes, or goes into your body, too quickly, with an effect similar to sugar. Blended smoothies have the best of both worlds. They have fiber, but it's digestible. And because of the fiber, the vegetables metabolize more slowly than they do in a juice, so blended smoothies are even healthier for you. That's why we recommend them—even in stage one of The Diet—over juices.

Blended smoothies are great for individuals of all ages (even older babies), since many people simply cannot digest raw foods like nuts and seeds and yes, even vegetables. When you blend a bunch of vegetables together in a powerful blender like the VitaMix or the Blendtec and create a *smoothie*, you're really eating the raw vegetables in their whole form, obtaining all their nutrients, enzymes, and fiber. In other words, blended smoothies allow you to obtain all the benefits of raw vegetables in a delicious drinkable form.

FERMENTED JUICES: We often use the VitaMix to blend a vegetable or several vegetables (such as celery, cabbage, and beets) in lots of water and then add Body Ecology's Cultured Vegetable Starter into the mixture. We then "culture" this veggie blend for 24 hours. Once it is fermented, we strain it, if necessary, and then refrigerate. We end up with a pretty extraordinary cultured "juice." Yes, beets are sweet, but they ferment beautifully, as the microflora gobble up the sugar in them. Beets help cleanse the liver.

To learn more about green smoothies and to download recipes, go to: **www.BodyEcology.com.**

Don't forget to download a copy of our **Quick Start Guide** at the same time.

☙

Notes

[16] Body Ecology ferments the kale and spinach we use in our Vitality SuperGreen so they do not suppress the thyroid.

Chapter 14

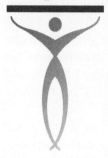

Body Ecology's Cultured Foods

We now present two of The Diet's special, signature foods—"super" foods that contribute immensely to healing and building your inner ecosystem: first, raw cultured vegetables; and second, kefir from the water of young green coconuts.

Raw cultured vegetables have been around for thousands of years, but we have never needed them more than we do today. Rich in lactobacilli and enzymes, alkaline-forming, and loaded with vitamins, they are an ideal food that can and should be consumed with every meal.

Since cultured vegetables are an excellent source of vitamin C, Dutch seamen used to carry them to prevent scurvy. For centuries, the Chinese have cultured cabbage each fall to ensure a source of greens through the winter (when they lacked refrigeration). Cultured vegetables are a favorite food of the long-lived Hunzas. Yogurt ads lead us to believe that eating yogurt ensures a long life, but it's really the active cultures of friendly bacteria (lactobacilli) inside it that are responsible for good health. Similarly, the enzymes and the high lactic acid in raw cultured vegetables promote wellness and longevity.

Cultured veggies taste tangy. It may be a new taste for you, but you will soon feel that no meal is complete without them. Even better, since they are all-vegetable, they combine with either a protein or a starch meal. They are slightly to the expansive end of the Expansion/Contraction Continuum, so they help balance the contractive nature of animal foods and sea salt.

So what exactly *are* raw cultured vegetables?

They're *sauerkraut*. The Austrians coined this word, from *sauer* (sour) and *kraut* (greens or plants). But we call them raw cultured vegetables, because we don't want you to mistake them for the salted and pasteurized sauerkraut sold in supermarkets and even some health-food stores. That kind of sauerkraut is definitely not on The Diet, because it is pasteurized. The pasteurization (heating) process destroys precious enzymes, and the added salt eliminates any health benefits. We'll teach you how to make these delicious raw cultured vegetables without heat or preservatives.

Benefits

- Raw cultured vegetables help reestablish your inner ecosystem. Their friendly bacteria are a less expensive alternative to probiotics (although we recommend both as you begin The Diet).

- They improve digestion. Knowing the benefits of raw foods, you may have decided to include raw vegetables with each meal. Yet when you begin The Diet, your digestive tract may be too weak to tolerate them. Cultured vegetables eliminate this concern, since they are already pre-digested. This means that even before they enter your mouth, the friendly bacteria have already converted the natural sugars and starches in the vegetables into lactic acid, a job your own saliva and digestive enzymes would do anyway. The enzymes in the cultured vegetables also help the digestion of other foods eaten with them.

- They increase longevity. You could think of the friendly bacteria in raw cultured vegetables as little enzyme powerhouses. By eating the vegetables, you will maintain your own enzyme reserve and use it to eliminate toxins, rejuvenate your cells, and strengthen your immune system—which all adds up to a longer, healthier life.

- They control cravings. Homemade cultured vegetables are ideal for appetite control and thus weight control. The veggies help take away cravings for the sweet taste in pastries, colas, bread, pasta, dairy, fruit, and other expansive foods not on The Diet.

- They are ideal for pregnant and nursing women. Pregnant women should eat cultured vegetables to ensure that their ecosystems are rich in friendly bacteria. They also help alleviate morning sickness during the early part of the pregnancy. Once the baby is born, the mother should continue eating these vegetables and drinking their juice. And the liquid from the cultured vegetables can be fed to the baby in tiny spoonfuls to relieve colic.

- They are alkaline and very cleansing. Cultured vegetables help restore balance if your body is in a toxic, acidic condition. Because they do trigger cleansing, you may have an increase in gas initially as the vegetables stir up waste and toxins in the intestinal tract. Soon, however, you will notice an improvement in your stools. To ease the discomfort of the gas, colonics and enemas are very useful during this period.

How to Make Cultured Veggies

Cultured vegetables are made by shredding cabbage or a combination of cabbage and other vegetables and then packing it tightly into an airtight container, left to ferment at room temperature for several days or longer. Friendly bacteria naturally present in the vegetables quickly lower the pH, making a more acidic environment so the bacteria can reproduce. The vegetables become soft, delicious, and somewhat "pickled."

The airtight container can be glass or stainless steel. Use a 1- to 1 1/2-quart container that seals with a rubber or plastic ring and a clamp-down lid. Room temperature means 70 degrees F. While three days is the minimum, we prefer to let ours sit for at least six or seven days, and have even left them culturing for weeks. You can taste them at different stages and decide for yourself.

In the winter months if your kitchen temperature falls below 70 degrees, wrap the container in a towel and place it inside an insulated or thermal chest. In the summer months the veggies culture faster. They may be ready in just three or four days.

During this fermentation period, the friendly bacteria are having a heyday, reproducing and converting sugars and starches to lactic acid. Once the initial process is over, it is time to slow down the bacterial activity by putting the cultured veggies in the refrigerator. The cold greatly slows the fermentation but does not stop it completely. Even if the veggies sit in your refrigerator for months, they will not spoil; instead they become like fine wine: more delicious with time. Properly made, cultured vegetables have at least an eight-month shelf life.

While it is not necessary to add a "starter culture" to your vegetables, we recommend that you do so just to ensure that your vegetables begin fermenting with a hardy strain of beneficial bacteria. Body Ecology's Cultured Vegetable Starter contains a very robust bacterium called *Lb. plantarum*.

Enjoying the Fruits of Your Labor

Once you master the basic technique, be creative. Try different vegetable combinations, and include dark green leafy vegetables like kale and collards. Soak, drain, and chop up some ocean vegetables, like dulse, wakame, hijiki, and arame. Add your favorite herbs (dried or fresh), seeds (dill or caraway), and juniper berries. Even lemon juice can be added to the "brine." Try leaving out the cabbage altogether and making a batch of cultured daikon.

I (Donna) have a friend, Cynthia Hamilton, who lives in Los Angeles and teaches classes on how to make cultured vegetables. She also sells them, calling them a "probiotic salad." Cynthia recently surprised me with a new recipe using kohlrabi, celery, garlic, ginger, and a green apple. It tastes wonderful! Don't be afraid of the little bit of sugar in the green apple. The microflora use it for food. The sugar will be long gone before you eat the cultured veggies. (If you create a great new recipe that you want to share with others on the B.E.D. around the world, please write or e-mail us and we will happily post it on our website.)

You may be thinking that making cultured veggies amounts to a big hassle. Well, it is possible to buy them commercially (see our Shopping List), but store-bought varieties come in smaller sizes and can be too costly for many people. You wouldn't be getting the "therapeutic amounts" you reap by making your own. So here's a suggestion: Plan a "CV Party" with your family and friends. Gather on a weekend afternoon to laugh together while you chop and pack the veggies. Make sure everyone leaves with enough containers to last until the next party. You and your loved ones will enjoy many meals incorporating one of the most medicinal and economical foods you'll ever eat.

Tips for Eating Raw Cultured Vegetables

Include at least 1/2 cup of the veggies in any meal where you are eating a protein or starch. Use the juice in salad dressing as a replacement for apple cider vinegar or lemon juice. You can also toss the veggies into salads, wrap them up in blue cornmeal tortillas, or serve them with crunchy blue corn chips.

Never heat the veggies, or the valuable enzymes and bacteria will be killed. If you leave them out at room temperature for a while, they come alive and start to multiply quickly. So sometimes when you open a jar, the veggies overflow and start bubbling out the top. This is good! It just means your batch is rich with viable bacteria ready to go to work in your digestive tract and establish a new inner ecology.

Two of Our Beginners' Recipes

One important secret to making really delicious yet medicinal cultured veggies is to use freshly harvested, organic, well-cleaned vegetables. After washing the veggies, spin them dry. Clean equipment is essential. Rinse everything you use in very hot water.

Version 1

3 heads green cabbage, shredded in a food processor
1 bunch kale, chopped by hand
(optional): 2 cups wakame ocean vegetables (measured after soaking), drained and chopped, with spine removed
1 Tbsp. dill seed

Version 2

3 heads green cabbage, shredded in a food processor
6 carrots, large, shredded in a food processor
3-inch piece ginger, peeled and chopped
6 cloves garlic, peeled and chopped

To Make Cultured Vegetables:

1. Combine all ingredients in a large bowl.

2. Remove several cups of this mixture and put into a blender.

3. Add enough filtered water to make a "brine" with the consistency of a thick juice. Blend well and then add brine back into first mixture. Stir well. (If using starter culture, see below.)

4. Pack mixture down into a glass or stainless-steel, air-tight container. Use your fist, a wooden dowel, or a potato masher to pack veggies tightly.

5. Fill container almost full, but leave about 2 inches of room at the top for veggies to expand.

6. Roll up several cabbage leaves into a tight "log" and place them on top to fill the remaining 2-inch space. Clamp jar closed.

7. Let veggies sit at room temperature for at least three days. A week is even better. Refrigerate to slow down fermentation. Enjoy!

To Use Body Ecology's Culture Starter:

Dissolve one package of starter culture in 1/4 cup warm (90° F) water. Add a small amount of sugar to feed the starter (try Rapadura, Sucanat, honey, agave nectar, or Body Ecology's EcoBloom™). Let starter/sugar mixture sit for about 20 minutes or longer while the *L. plantarum* and other bacteria "wake up" and begin feeding on the sugar. Add this starter culture to the brine (step 3).

Body Ecology's Newest Super Food: Young Green Coconuts

Great discoveries often stem from a touch of serendipity and some creative experimentation. Don Kidson, owner of the Living Lighthouse (the raw foods center for the Los Angeles area), introduced me (Donna) to the value of young green coconuts. Most Americans have seen and tasted the milk and meat of the mature (brown, hairy) coconut; a green coconut is really the same food, but it is just younger. Sometimes the green outer shells are cut off before they are shipped to US markets. Look for either the green shell or a white "husk" if the outer shell has been removed. You may not see them in the produce section of your big-chain supermarket, but they are readily available in Asian, Latin, and other ethnic or farmers' markets. Many health-food stores will carry them upon request.

Although the liquid of the young coconut has an abundance of B vitamins and minerals, I knew that it was too sweet to be medicinal. Drinking it would make the blood too acidic and would encourage the growth of pathogens and cancers. The idea of adding Body Ecology's Kefir Starter to this liquid and "culturing it" kept popping into my mind. I knew it would be a perfect medium for the growth of beneficial microflora.

On a pretty summer night in Malibu, Don, two close friends, and I combined the starter and coconut water, let it rest for 24 hours, and were delighted with what we had created. All the sugar disappeared and a fizzy, sour, champagne-like drink, like a spritzer, was born. Don and I began teaching many people how to duplicate this great new discovery, and the results were miraculous.

What People Say about Coconut Water Kefir

1. It completely stops your cravings for sugar. Imagine the benefits!

2. It aids digestion of all foods.

3. It has a "toning" effect on the intestines, even flattening the abdomen!

4. It appears to cleanse the liver. In Chinese medicine the liver rules the skin, eyes, and joints. Coconut water kefir eases aches and joint pains. Many people report having a prettier complexion. They experience the brown liver spots on the skin fading away and skin tags, moles, or warts drying up and disappearing. Vision also improves.

5. It contains high levels of valuable minerals, including potassium, natural sodium, calcium, and magnesium, which explains why the hair, skin, and nails become stronger and have a prettier shine.

6. It appears to have a beneficial, cleansing effect on the endocrine system (adrenals, thyroid, pituitary, and ovaries). Women find they have easier periods; some who had experienced early menopause have found this important monthly cleansing returning again.

7. It increases energy and gives you an overall feeling of good health.

Young green coconuts yield several delicious foods. You can ferment the water (not "coconut milk") into that delicious, healing kefir. You can also eat the very special meat. Soft and pudding-like, this meat is high in protein, enzyme-rich, and very easy to digest. Like all seeds and nuts, coconut is a protein fat, but this seed provides an excellent source of lauric and caprylic fatty acids. You can scoop the meat out of the shell and eat it raw, but we recommend you ferment it since it has too much sugar (see instructions on next page). When you ferment the meat, you'll have a sort of kefir "cheese," a fabulous fermented base for salad dressings and dips; or just eat it plain as is. It's like eating yogurt, only it's dairy free. Enjoy it as a creamy pudding by sweetening it with stevia and a favorite flavoring.

How to Crack Those Coconuts

First, remove the 1–11/2 cups of water inside the young coconut and use it to make kefir. To do this, begin by resting a Phillips-head screwdriver on the pointed head of the coconut. Pound it several times with a hammer until you break through the coconut shell, making a hole. Rout out this hole to make it bigger. Repeat this step again, making another hole near the first. Then twirl the coconut around and make a third hole opposite the other two. Now flip the coconut over onto a glass jar or 2-cup Pyrex measuring cup and let the water drain.

Use the water from about 3 coconuts with 1 package of starter. Warm the water slightly to approximately 90 degrees. Pour warmed coconut water into a glass jar and add starter culture. We recommend you use Body Ecology's Kefir Starter, which contains both lactobacillus and friendly yeast to make your young coconut kefir. If you want acidophilus and bifidus bacteria in this beverage as well, simply add a package of Essential Duo Starter and increase the amount of coconut water (5–6 coconuts). Let the coconut water sit in a warm, stable environment (70 degrees) for 36 hours. You'll know it's done when the color changes to a milky white, and usually there's a bit of bubbling or foam on top. This means that most of the sugar has been fermented out by the microflora. When you drink, make sure it tastes tart and tangy. This is another sign that all the sugar is gone. I swear by this wonderful new kefir. I wouldn't be without it, despite my busy schedule. Its medicinal benefits are well worth the time it takes to make it!

Special Notes: You can use about 1/4 cup from your first half gallon to "transfer" the friendly bacteria to your next half gallon of kefir. Do this up to seven times with one package of starter. Your second batch of kefir will only take 24 hours to ferment since the microflora are now "awake" and will start working upon the sugars immediately. It's best to always warm the liquid to about 90 degrees before adding the starter so that the microflora wake up quickly and begin to feed on the sugar. Then place the glass jar into an insulated container so it will maintain a steady temperature of about 70 degrees while fermenting.

Getting to the delicious white spoon-meat inside the coconut takes more effort, but it too ferments into a delicious soft "pudding" or "cheese" in about 8 hours. We suggest you use a Chinese cleaver and a hammer to split the coconut shell, then take a spoon and remove the soft meat. Wash off any brown shell and place the spoon-meat into a blender with enough water to make a creamy smooth pudding. Add several tablespoons of the already-fermented coconut kefir water to the pureed spoon-meat or use culture starter, and let your pudding sit out at 70 degrees for 8 hours to ferment.

Ways to Enjoy Coconut Water Kefir

Remember, since you now have two more cultured foods in your healing arsenal, you can devise many different ways to eat them. A half cup of the coconut water kefir with meals greatly helps digestion. You can add ginger, stevia, lemon, and/or lime if desired. A half cup at bedtime will help establish a healthy inner ecosystem. Studies from Europe show that when you are lying still during sleep, the microflora reproduce faster. In the morning, combine a half cup of the young coconut water with unsweetened cranberry or black currant juice as a great wake-up tonic. And in stage two of The Diet when you start introducing a little fruit for breakfast, the coconut kefir microflora will happily enjoy the sugar in the fruit and leave you with its vitamins and minerals.

If you are lactose intolerant because you do not have dairy-loving microflora thriving in your inner ecosystem, begin adding them by drinking the coconut water kefir and eating young coconut kefir "cheese." Then slowly introduce organic milk kefir (the subject of the next chapter), gradually increasing the amount, and you will soon find yourself enjoying dairy kefir as well.

☙

Chapter 15

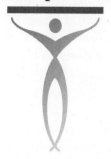

The Magic of Kefir

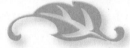

Since the first printing of this book, thousands of people around the world have discovered for themselves the benefits of the Body Ecology Diet. We have received hundreds of letters attesting to this, and are very grateful to know that so many of you are becoming well. Many of you have reported so much improvement that you call yourselves "cured." Some of you are symptom free; others tell us that they immediately feel better, but that their symptoms return when they stop following The Diet. And for a significant number of you, digestive problems persist or there is unwanted weight loss. This means that the inner ecosystem still is not fully reestablished and needs some additional help. It also means that even the healthiest foods may be passing through your body without their nutrients being adequately absorbed.

If that's the case, the solution is to continue your healing process and intensify your focus on restoring the integrity of your inner ecosystem as quickly as possible so your digestive tract can begin to assimilate food properly. Remember, you are not completely well until your inner ecosystem is restored.

Without detracting from the importance of The Body Ecology Diet, probiotics, Vitality SuperGreen, cultured vegetables, and fermented young coconut foods, we would now like to introduce you to kefir . . . a wonderful ancient food that we believe will help many of you enter the final phase of getting well, restore the integrity of your digestive tract, and add to the effectiveness of everything else you've done so far.

Donna's Story

Many years ago, I was introduced to kefir, but did not understand or appreciate its value. An excellent colon therapist had mentioned to me that kefir, especially goat milk kefir, has a very beneficial, toning effect on the colon. After a bit of searching, I found a goat farmer and master cheese maker in Pennsylvania who made delicious kefir. I ordered some and tried it, but was highly skeptical since it was made from milk, which sent up a red flag for me. Milk is mucus-forming; feeds yeast; and in Chinese medicine, produces a sticky, "damp" quality. Besides, I had always been lactose intolerant and allergic to milk. So, even though I enjoyed it, I quickly dismissed kefir as an unimportant food.

Then, as always happens for me, I began to see signs that I needed to open my mind to new possibilities. For example, I happened to turn on the television (which I rarely watch) and saw a program about fish in a Canadian lake that produced mucus to protect themselves as the lake's pH level rose due to acid rain. Several days later, I lunched with a friend whose daughter had brought home a book describing how a fish had totally covered itself with mucus when it washed up on the beach, protecting itself until the rising tide returned it safely back to sea. I realized mucus can be a protection. After a little more reflection, I remembered that all things in this universe have both a positive and a negative side and I had been focusing only on the negative aspect of mucus.

I tucked this information away in my mind, and as I began collecting more information about kefir, more parts of the puzzle fell into place. For example, I knew that at birth, a newborn has no inner ecosystem and must establish it during the first few months of life. Nature decrees that mother's milk be available for all offspring of mammals. This milk lays down a bed of clean mucus, allowing friendly bacteria to establish themselves. Breast milk is an excellent source of protective agents such as lauric acid, a powerful antimicrobial that deactivates pathogenic bacteria, yeast, fungi, and some viruses. This protects the baby until the inner ecosystem is well established with positive bacteria and its immune system matures.

As I began to add up all the facts, I realized that: 1) there is both good, clean-quality mucus and toxic mucus; 2) good mucus coats and protects the interior lining of the digestive tract; and 3) unlike yeast, which burrow into the intestinal walls with their tentacles, good bacteria do not have tentacles and must be caught by this clean mucus, where they nestle into their warm, acidic environment, fed by the sugar (lactose) in mother's milk. Mucus, I finally had to admit, was an essential part of a healthy inner ecosystem.

People with candidiasis have a very unhealthy inner ecosystem. They have an overgrowth of fungus or yeast, and very toxic bowels. In order to heal, they must first cleanse the colon and control the yeast overgrowth. Then they must reestablish an inner ecosystem teeming with beneficial bacteria. At this second stage, a sufferer of candidiasis could be compared to a newborn babe . . . both must have this vibrant, living inner world if they are going to assimilate nutrients; create a strong immune system; and live a long, fruitful life.

It was becoming clearer to me that kefir had tremendous healing power. With its laxative effect, it helped clean my colon. Its beneficial bacteria and yeast helped control the pathogenic yeast and repopulate my colon with a favorable, new life force. And kefir, being cultured, was much healthier than milk.

In ancient times, kefir was given to the people of the Caucasus region of Eurasia as a gift from the gods. Perhaps these "gods" were watching over mankind and offering us this miracle food at a time when we desperately needed it. Now, if only I could learn to make kefir and test out my theory. The problem was that no one had grains or a starter culture, there was almost no information available, and the few people who knew about kefir did not want to share their "secrets." Then a miracle happened!

After the publication of the first edition of *The Body Ecology Diet*, I felt drawn to take a spiritual sabbatical to recharge myself and give thanks for the success of the book. I traveled to a sacred area of Japan and attended a ceremony honoring the creation of humanity. A friend from Sendai, Japan, joined me the evening before the ceremony and brought with him Mrs. Kwai, a woman I had never met before. He told me that his friend had felt very strongly compelled to come and bring with her something she thought I needed. Amazingly, it was a little brown pot of kefir grains cultivating in milk. Mrs. Kwai opened the container and, with her strainer and a spoon, showed me how to make kefir.

My prayers were being answered. In amazement I brought the kefir back to my room, still not fully appreciating what I had been given. I ate the kefir, loved the taste, and felt a surge of strength after my tiring journey.

When I returned home, everything started coming together. I began making kefir every day. At first I was skeptical, as I always am about new foods, so I told no one about it. Each morning I had a glass of it, and within two weeks couldn't believe how much energy I had. When you are over 50 (as I am), if you eat the wrong foods, it shows and you look your age. However, I was amazed that each day I seemed to look younger. Others noticed it, too, and kept telling me how good I looked. Any woman loves that.

One day, I received a call from a woman who was using alternative methods, including the Body Ecology principles, to heal herself from non-Hodgkin's lymphoma. Yes, the lab reports showed no trace of cancer, but I could still hear a weakness in her voice. Intuitively, I knew the kefir would help her.

It did! She called again two weeks later and the change in her voice was remarkable. She said she was feeling much, much better. From that day on I recommended kefir to many more people.

Women with vaginal yeast infections told me that kefir cleared up the infection. Young women with eating disorders and people with Crohn's disease, stomach problems, ulcers, diverticulitis, depression, and constipation all reported that they were becoming well, simply by following The Diet and having kefir for their breakfast meal.

Thousands of people are now on the Body Ecology Diet. They have been spreading the word about it and about kefir, too. Many are making kefir at home and love to do so. (Later, we'll tell you how.)

I can't recommend kefir highly enough. It is a nutritious, incredibly delicious food. If your body is ready for it and you find you tolerate it well, kefir can be essential to your achieving maximum health and immunity. As you read this book and begin to drink kefir, you'll realize, too, that it is an ancient remedy for modern maladies: a true gift from heaven. Enjoy!

What Is Kefir?

Kefir is a cultured and microbial-rich food that helps restore the body's inner ecology. It contains strains of beneficial yeast and beneficial bacteria (in a symbiotic relationship) that give it antibiotic properties. A natural antibiotic—and it is made from milk! The finished product is not unlike that of a drinking-style yogurt, but kefir has a more tart, refreshing taste and is more medicinal.

The Body Ecology Diet recommends avoiding dairy products because they contain a milk sugar called lactose that feeds yeast and creates mucus. But kefir does *not* feed yeast, and it usually doesn't even bother people who are lactose intolerant. That's because the friendly bacteria and the beneficial yeast growing in the kefir consume most of the lactose and provide very efficient enzymes (lactase) for consuming whatever lactose is still left after the culturing process. Yes, kefir is mucus-forming, but only slightly so if you follow some simple food-combining rules (more on these later).

And here's the capper: the slightly mucus-forming quality is exactly what makes kefir work for us. The mucus has a "clean" quality to it that coats the lining of the digestive tract, creating a sort of nest where beneficial bacteria can settle and colonize. This makes the other probiotics you may be taking even more potent: they now have a better chance to take hold and proliferate in your intestines, helping you really "get your money's worth." By the way, kefir can be made from any type of milk, including cow's milk, goat's milk, or soy milk.

Kefir was traditionally made from gelatinous white or yellow particles called "grains." The grains contain the bacteria/yeast mixture clumped together with casein (milk protein) and polysaccharides (complex sugars). They look like pieces of coral or small clumps of cauliflower and range from the size of a grain of wheat to that of a hazelnut. Some grains have been known to grow in large flat sheets that can be big enough to cover your hand. No other milk culture forms grains or has beneficial yeast . . . making kefir truly unique. Once the grains have fermented the milk by incorporating their friendly organisms into the final product, you should remove them with a strainer before drinking the kefir. The grains can then be rinsed and added to a new batch of milk, and the process continues indefinitely.

Kefir grains are a little more difficult to work with since they can be contaminated easily when they are rinsed and transferred into fresh milk. Also, since you cannot see the lactobacillus and yeast colonizing on the grains, you cannot be certain that *the* correct microflora are there. In other words, if the lactobacilli crowded out the yeast—as they sometimes aggressively do—you wouldn't know it. And while you would still have a fermented drink, it would not be kefir. For these reasons, Body Ecology now offers a "starter" made from grains and composed of lactobacillus and two especially hardy strains of yeast. A starter is just that—a starter that allows you to "start" a quart of kefir. From that original quart, you can then make much larger quantities of kefir. (Our Body Ecology starters come with easy-to-follow instructions and are available at fine health-food stores, or by calling 1-866-4BE-DIET.)

Kefir vs. Yogurt

Kefir, experts believe, has more nutritive value than yogurt. Its very active yeast and bacteria excel in digesting the foods you eat and in keeping the environment of the colon clean and healthy.

Yogurt is made by adding a starter culture to milk and gently heating it to a certain temperature. To make kefir, you must start with the grains or a starter, and no heating is required. This means that if you can obtain a reliable source of fresh, raw milk, you can retain enzymes that would normally be destroyed by the heat of pasteurization. Kefir "cultures" at room temperature in approximately 16 to 24 hours, right on your kitchen counter.

After your inner ecology is restored, you may find that you now digest yogurt well and want to make use of its friendly bacteria. But choose kefir first. Its friendly bacteria and yeast are crucial to the restoration process. We think of them as a

SWAT team moving in quickly to begin the therapeutic process, efficiently doing the job they were created to do.

You may see a product in the store that claims to be kefir, but read the label carefully. Unless it has strains of friendly bacteria and the good yeast, it is most likely a drinkable yogurt.

Benefits of Friendly Bacteria

With more than 400 different species of beneficial microorganisms living inside a healthy gut, why not give them the optimal environment? As we've said, kefir lays down a foundation of clean mucus so these beneficial organisms have a place to thrive. When you add probiotics (friendly organisms purchased from your health-food store), they too will find a receptive home much more quickly if a favorable environment has already been created.

You can easily make kefir fresh every day or so in your own kitchen so that its friendly yeast and bacteria are readily available to do their job in your intestinal tract.

After you restore the balance to your inner ecology using the Body Ecology Diet, cultured vegetables, young coconut kefir and kefir cheese, probiotics, and cow- or goat-milk kefir, your intestinal tract will be teeming with friendly organisms. Then you will be better able to enjoy some foods containing natural sugars (fruits, whole cereal grains, and the sweeter vegetables such as yams and parsnips), and you may tolerate that occasional binge on really sugary food such as a piece of cake or candy. The beneficial bacteria gobble up the sugar for themselves first, leaving little to carry into the rest of your body. Of course, we are not endorsing foods with refined sugar, but it certainly doesn't hurt to be prepared and "well armed." Ironically, when you eat cultured foods, you will lose your cravings for carbohydrates and sugars.

If you are a parent worried about all the sugary foods your child wants (and often gets), kefir is especially useful for establishing and maintaining a strong immune system. To make a kefir treat that kids love, add the natural, sweet-tasting herb stevia; some non-alcoholic fruit flavorings; or vanilla. You can even freeze this mixture and make frozen kefir popsicles (some microflora will die when frozen).

All cultured foods, including kefir, keep the small and large intestines clean and free of parasites. Once in the large intestine, the beneficial bacteria create lactic acid that balances the pH level there. In this acidic environment, parasites and other unfriendly organisms cannot survive. Kefir's beneficial yeast and bacteria are ready to ambush any parasite eggs or larvae before they have a chance to establish themselves and multiply.

With its .02% alcohol content (produced by the yeast), kefir is acidic when you make it; yet it becomes alkaline-forming in the body once you eat it. This means that the overall quality of the blood remains slightly more alkaline and you remain healthy.

The friendly bacteria and yeast in kefir provide a good advance team for other probiotic cultures like acidophilus and bifidus. Kefir "clears the land" and establishes clean, healthy sites for new colonies of friendly bacteria. When the new settlers arrive (the friendly bacteria you buy in your health-food store or generate internally by eating cultured foods), they remain and thrive, ensuring a far better return on your investment.

New research has found that stomach ulcers are often caused by pathogenic bacteria called *Helicobacter pylori*. Expensive antibiotic therapy is now being used to kill this invader. Kefir may prevent such ulcers. Remember that antibiotics kill all bacteria, both the good and the bad, so it is important to remain on the Body Ecology Diet if you must take antibiotics, using cultured vegetables, the coconut and dairy kefir, and probiotics to rebuild your inner ecosystem.

We have found both kinds of kefir to be beneficial in cases of diarrhea, which is common in those afflicted with AIDS or in cancer patients undergoing chemotherapy or radiation.

Nutritional Benefits

Kefir from milk is a complete protein with all the essential amino acids. By the time you drink kefir, its friendly bacteria have already partially digested the protein, making it much easier for *you* to digest. High amounts of protein are critical to healing, and your body must have adequate minerals in order to assimilate the protein. Kefir provides these, too. Both milk kefir and young coconut kefir contain an abundance of calcium and magnesium.

Tryptophan, an essential amino acid found in milk kefir, combines with the calcium and magnesium to help calm the nervous system. Some people call kefir "nature's tranquilizer" or "nature's Prozac." Its calming effect is great for people who are high-strung or nervous, for hyperactive children, or for people with sleep disorders, such as the elderly. The body converts tryptophan into serotonin, an important chemical known as a *neurotransmitter*. Balanced serotonin levels can cure depression and constipation, induce sleep, and prevent waking during the night. This conversion is helped along by vitamin B-6, which is also abundant in kefir.

Kefir also has ample phosphorus, the second-most-abundant mineral in our bodies. Phosphorus is important in utilizing carbohydrates, fats, and proteins for growth, cell maintenance, and energy. A phosphorus deficiency can result in the loss of appetite.

Kefir and the B Vitamins

People with candidiasis are usually deficient in the B vitamins and in vitamin K because the body's use of these vitamins depends on adequate levels of friendly bacteria in the intestinal tract. When kefir is included in the diet, your body should soon be able to manufacture sufficient amounts of these needed bacteria. Vitamin K promotes blood clotting, encourages the flow of urine, relieves menstrual cramps, increases vitality and longevity, and enhances liver functioning.

Kefir provides biotin, another B vitamin, which is missing in people with candidiasis. Biotin is a coenzyme that assists in the manufacture of fatty acids and in the oxidation of fatty acids and carbohydrates. Without biotin, the body's production of essential fatty acids is impaired. Biotin also aids in the body's assimilation of protein and other B vitamins: folic acid, pantothenic acid, and B-12. A deficiency of biotin can cause muscular pain, poor appetite, dry skin, lack of energy, or depression and a distressed nervous system.

Kefir is an excellent source of vitamin B-12, which is essential for longevity. It is the only vitamin that contains essential mineral elements. It cannot be made synthetically but must be grown, like penicillin, in bacteria or molds. B-12 is necessary for the normal metabolism of nerve tissue and for red blood cell formation. B-12 builds immunity and has been used to increase energy and counteract allergens. It is also required for normal growth and is important for fertility and during pregnancy. Plus, it works along with folic acid, another member of the B complex, in facilitating the synthesis of choline, a fat and cholesterol dissolver that plays an important role in the transmission of nerve impulses. Choline also helps regulate kidney, liver, and gallbladder function and aids in the prevention of gallstones.

B-12 helps the assimilation of vitamin A into body tissues by aiding carotene absorption, or *conversion*. It also aids in the production of DNA and RNA, the body's genetic material. B-12 needs to be combined with calcium during absorption to benefit the body properly; nature has provided for that in kefir.

Kefir is rich in thiamin (vitamin B-1), also known as the "morale vitamin" because of its beneficial effects on the nervous system and on mental attitude. Thiamin is linked with enhanced learning capacity; growth in children; and improvement in the muscle tone of the stomach, intestines, and heart. It is essential for stabilizing the appetite and improving digestion, particularly of carbohydrates, sugar, and alcohol.

Kefir from cow's milk is a wonderful source of folic acid (recommended for pregnant women to prevent spinal deformities in their unborn children).

Benefits to Your Overall Health

Kefir helps stop food cravings because the body feels nourished as an inner balance is achieved and nutritional deficiencies are corrected.

Kefir provides a "sour" taste. Chinese medicine teaches us there are five tastes necessary for balance in the body; the sour one is not commonly found in our American diet.

The skin prospers from kefir. It will become moist and creamy and, over time, you will notice a refinement of the pores. You can use kefir externally to help moisturize your skin; yet, it is beneficial for oily skin, too. Fermented milks contain lactic acid, which is one of the naturally occurring alpha hydroxy acids (AHA) so popular in the cosmetic world today.

Kefir is cooling to the body, so it is ideal to consume when you have a fever or any other condition resulting in body heat such as a herpes outbreak or AIDS.

After taking antibiotics, kefir is very useful for reestablishing friendly bacteria in the intestines. Kefir is "nature's antibiotic."

Using it helps reduce the need for antibiotics in the future.

Kefir's friendly bacteria automatically show up in the vagina, or you can implant them more directly as a douche.

While colonic therapy helps cleanse pathogenic yeast from the large intestine, such yeast colonize in the small intestine as well. Fermented foods have a cleansing effect on both intestines. Once these are free of pathogens and colonized with beneficial microorganisms, the liver is able to function much better as well.

Both young coconut kefir and milk kefir help produce more pleasant breath, healthier bowel movements, and sweeter-smelling stools. And they will eventually help eliminate flatulence!

How to Introduce Kefir into Your Diet

Some people thrive on kefir from milk right from the start, and others may need to proceed more slowly. People with candidiasis have a leaky, permeable gut lining. This lining must be healed before you can start drinking kefir made from dairy. It's essential that the protein in milk kefir (casein) does not leak through the gut lining and cause further problems, including allergies. (NOTE: Young coconut kefir and kefir cheese have no caseins, and are allowed in the early stages of The Diet. They introduce dairy-loving bacteria into the intestines so that when you eventually drink kefir made from milk, you'll digest it easily.)

Once your leaky, permeable gut has healed (8 to 12 weeks on The Diet), start with about four ounces in the morning on an empty stomach. Every week increase the amount until you are able to drink more.

The Body Ecology Diet was developed for people who have a problem with a "leaky," inflamed mucosal lining; and Vitality SuperGreen has ingredients that nourish the lining as well. Cultured vegetables, young coconut kefir, and the other fermented foods we recommend will become important tools for creating healthy intestines.

Moreover, people with candidiasis have what Chinese medicine calls the condition of dampness. Unfermented and improperly combined dairy products can lead to even more dampness and excess mucus. Here are some suggestions for introducing kefir while conquering dampness:

- Eat Body Ecology Diet foods, which will help heal a leaky gut and have a "drying" effect.

- Use proper food-combining techniques to make kefir less mucus-forming (see below).

- Drink plenty of water, and eat grains that have been soaked and then cooked. These add moisture and fiber to the colon.

- Clean your colon. If a colon is free of blockages, kefir is tolerated more quickly. We have found that people who report having trouble with kefir often have not followed the advice on colon cleansing. You probably also need to add a significant amount of acidophilus and bifidus bacteria to your small and large intestines. These wonderful bacteria help clean and improve the health of your entire digestive tract.

- Be sure to get adequate exercise. Exercise stimulates the colon and improves elimination.

- Make your kefir from goat's milk if you find cow's milk is mucus-forming. The milk from a mother's breast is alkaline-forming. Goat's milk is also alkaline, while cow's milk is acidic. This could explain why goat's milk is often better tolerated by some people. It also has more calcium, magnesium, phosphorus, and potassium than cow's milk. Goat's milk contains no folic acid, however, so pregnant and nursing mothers should consider a folic acid supplement and eat leafy greens, broccoli, root vegetables, and whole grains. (Goat's milk will also require more starter culture.) It is naturally homogenized, so the fat cannot be separated. If your digestion of fats is poor at this time, you may do better on a non-fat, or low-fat, cow's milk kefir where the fat floats to the top and is easily separated. Raw cow's *or* goat's milk is much more easily digested than pasteurized.

Food-Combining Rules for Kefir

Make kefir with the freshest milk possible (raw is best), then add:

- Raw or lightly steamed vegetables (try a salad with our kefir dressing recipe, or use our recipe to make a kefir dip for raw veggies)

- Acid (sour) fruits such as strawberries, lemons, limes, grapefruits, pineapples, cranberries, or blueberries

- Soaked nuts or seeds

Kefir smoothies are especially delicious and very popular as a breakfast for children. In the beginning the non-alcoholic flavorings work well, but as your child becomes well, you can add acid fruits. Simply blend kefir, your favorite berries or flavorings, and stevia. A little unrefined flax seed oil is a "must" for children . . . especially those with eczema and ADHD.

To ensure that kefir is not overly mucus-forming, do not combine it with animal proteins (nuts and seeds are fine) or starches.

Around the world, however, kefir is eaten throughout the day, even as a digestive aid after a meal. While we do not recommend this, see what works for you. Some people think that eating kefir about an hour before bedtime helps them relax and fall asleep. Remember, it is rich in tryptophan.

In the chapter on food combining, we recommended you wait three hours after eating dairy foods before dining on animal protein or starches. However, because kefir's protein is pre-digested and the friendly yeast and bacteria speed up digestion, you need only wait about 45 minutes to an hour before eating something else.

Kefir makes a great morning meal. It's a much better breakfast for American children than the traditional bowl of cereal or Pop-Tart.

Ingredients of a Spectacular Kefir Drink

Make your kefir with the freshest milk possible, then add as many of the following ingredients as you wish:

- Up to 1 Tbsp. of unrefined oil or oil blends, flax seed oil, roasted pumpkin seed, or Essential Woman (Barlean's).

- A pinch of sea salt . . . to balance out the fats and for alkaline balance.

- Lecithin granules to taste. Lecithin assists in the digestion of fat. If you make kefir from skim milk, the only fat will come from the unrefined oil. However, the beneficial microorganisms prefer a little fat, so 2% or whole milk makes a better-tasting kefir.

- Fiber (flax seed), acidophilus, bifidus, and Body Ecology's Eco Bloom (food for the friendly bacteria) would be excellent additions.

- Probiotics, if you are taking them currently.

- Natural flavorings or herbs, such as nutmeg, cinnamon, or non-alcoholic vanilla or fruit flavorings (peach, strawberry, lemon, lime, raspberry, orange, tangerine).

- Non-caloric sugar substitutes such as stevia.

Is Kefir Right for Me?

Some people believe that milk and dairy products should be eaten only by newborns, and that since no adult animals in the wild drink milk, we adult humans shouldn't either. Others have an ethical objection to dairy products. You need to decide for yourself.

Perhaps you will achieve such great results with kefir that you will want to continue on it indefinitely. Or you may want to use it for a short period of time, being mindful of its mucus-forming effects. Or maybe two to three times a week is best for you.

Studies show that cultured foods such as raw vegetables, kefir, or miso and tempeh in the more traditional Asian diet are key components in a genuinely healthy diet. It is wise to keep recolonizing the intestinal tract with beneficial bacteria from the day we are born to the day we draw our last breath. Research shows that beneficial bacteria disappear from the stool once probiotic products or foods are discontinued.

We would not recommend anything that we haven't found to be superior in helping people heal, but we also know how important it is to trust the wisdom of what your own body tells you. Learn to listen to its signs and signals.

A Word of Caution

Constipation

Even though kefir is traditionally recommended as a laxative, a small percentage of people find it constipating. This may be because they lack the enzymes necessary to digest the milk protein (casein) or the milk fats. Try making your kefir from non-fat, organic milk and taking enzymes (Body Ecology's ASSIST Dairy & Protein, pancreatin, or hydrochloric acid with pepsin). Milk is also slightly dehydrating. Try diluting four ounces of kefir with several ounces of water and drinking this small amount in the morning on an empty stomach.

Be sure to add other probiotics that thrive in the small intestine and colon, especially acidophilus and lactobacillus and various bifidus strains. Expect them to take two to three weeks to bring about an improvement. With time, more dairy-loving bacteria and yeast will colonize your digestive tract. Once this happens, you can digest dairy better.

A little-known fact you may find extremely useful is that serotonin, the brain chemical linked to mood, is actually manufactured principally in the gut. When your serotonin levels are low, depression and constipation occur (since serotonin also influences peristaltic movement).* Kefir, rich in tryptophan that converts into serotonin, has cured many of depression and constipation. However, when serotonin levels are too high, constipation will occur. Drinking too much kefir can slow peristaltic movement and may be the cause of constipation. Anti-depression drugs also cause constipation and other gut problems since they stop the gut from shutting down production of serotonin and allow too much of it to continually circulate in your bloodstream. *Kefir* in Turkish means to "feel good." Now you know why.

If you become constipated after adding kefir to your diet, ask yourself these questions:

- *Am I drinking enough mineral water?* Milk is dehydrating

- *Am I eating enough fiber?* Kefir lacks fiber, so be sure to eat plenty of the high-fiber foods: raw vegetables (fresh and cultured), salads, and the Body Ecology grains.

- *Am I following the food-combining rules?*

- *Am I drinking too much kefir and skipping other meals?* Since kefir is so delicious and is the perfect "fast food," it is easy to overindulge in it, skipping essential high-fiber meals.

- *Am I eating sugary foods and flour products?* Both are constipating.

- *Am I deficient in magnesium?* Milk is rich in calcium and phosphorus (for bone development) but only has a very small amount of magnesium (needed to assist in the assimilation of the other two minerals). Consuming a dairy food will increase calcium and phosphorus levels only, creating a greater calcium/magnesium imbalance. Deficiency in magnesium is a major cause of constipation. Increase your intake of magnesium-rich foods and even take magnesium supplements.

Teeth

A final reminder: brush your teeth after you eat or drink any milk product. The milk protein can cause plaque that can lead to decay (just as any food left in the mouth without proper rinsing and care can lead to decay).

Vitamin C

If you have a cold or other condition that creates a lot of mucus, such as an ear infection, stop your kefir and start taking therapeutic doses of vitamin C (several thousand milligrams per day, to bowel tolerance).

Where Can I Get Some Kefir?

Milk kefir made right in your own kitchen is not only delicious, it's economical and fun to make. You'll also have a choice of the quality and kind of milk to use. Choices include non-fat, 1%, 2%, or whole cow's milk; goat's milk; soy milk; and even raw milk (if available). The great news is that homemade kefir is also unbelievably easy. Just warm the milk, add the starter culture, shake or stir, then cover it and let it sit for 24 hours on your kitchen countertop. You'll know it is ready when the milk turns thick and you could stand a toothpick up in it. Then, shake your kefir briskly and refrigerate it to stop the fermentation process. If you leave it for several hours longer, it will start to turn into kefir cheese.

Of course, there are times when you may want to simply purchase your kefir. Carefully read the label to make sure a product labeled kefir is true kefir with yeast. Kefir produced by Helios Nutrition is the only kefir that carries our Body Ecology seal of approval. Helios Nutrition makes a wonderful, truly organic kefir with chicory inulin, a medium- and long-chain FOS** (food that encourages the growth of lactobacillus and bifidus microorganisms). The plain flavor (unsweetened) is the one to buy when you have candidiasis. Plain is delicious, but you can change the taste simply by adding one of the non-alcoholic flavorings with stevia found in your health-food store.***

Points to Remember about Kefir

• To obtain a microbial-rich, potent kefir, make a new batch every day or two. Use the freshest organic milk you can find to ensure high quality and good flavor.

• Kefir is the healthy equivalent of a "fast food." It provides a filling meal that is nutrient-rich and easy to digest. Its high liquid content makes it an ideal breakfast food, since it's best taken on an empty stomach.

• In Europe and Russia, babies begin drinking kefir diluted with water at four months of age. The Russians know that kefir helps build a strong immune system. Upon arriving at school, every child is offered a glass of plain kefir compliments of the government. Wouldn't it be wonderful if American schools and day-care centers were as savvy?

• If you are lactose intolerant, try kefir. The yeast and bacteria in kefir digest the milk sugar lactose. Any remaining is taken care of by the lactase enzymes. After reestablishing your inner ecosystem, you may find that you can more easily digest other dairy foods.

∾

Notes

* Read *The Second Brain: A Groundbreaking New Understanding of Nervous Disorders of the Stomach and Intestine,* by Dr. Michael Gershon.

** FOS feeds friendly bacteria and enhances calcium and magnesium absorption. Please be aware that short-chain FOS, commonly used in many products, feeds klebsiella and candida. Body Ecology and Helios Nutrition use chicory inulin Frutafit from Imperial Sensus, a medium- and long-chain FOS that is safe for candida.

***Kefir starter culture is available by calling 1-866-4BE-DIET. Helios Nutrition kefir is available in fine health-food stores, or by calling 1-888-3HELIOS.

Chapter 16

Cravings: How to Stay on The Diet

If you're like most people, you're accustomed to eating mostly what you want, when you want. Deciding to start the Body Ecology Diet requires many changes in your eating habits and even your lifestyle (you have to shop for new foods, probably at different stores, and cook them in new ways). It's very natural to start craving foods you have eliminated, and it's likely that the main craving you will have will be for a sweet taste: *anything* that has sugar or tastes sweet.

Sweet Dreams

Our desire for a sweet taste starts when we're born and can be better understood if we use the expansion/contraction principle. Breast milk, created to nourish both the baby and its developing inner ecosystem, is rich in milk sugar. An expanding food, it helps babies—who are contracted little beings—grow and expand. Baby's first foods, pureed fruits and sweet vegetables (carrots, winter squash, sweet potatoes), are also expanding. This natural sugar is not a problem if a healthy inner ecosystem has been established and maintained.

The beneficial microflora thrive on it. But since a new mother is never taught to focus on her baby's inner world—that is, on creating a strong digestion/immune system—this rarely happens. Other foods are introduced, especially the many processed foods we eat today, and sugar in one form or another becomes part of most meals. By the time we are adults, we are completely unaware that we have had a sugar addiction since birth. When the Body Ecology Diet eliminates these all at once, no wonder we crave something sweet.

How to Satisfy That Sweet Tooth

The first three to five days on The Diet are the most difficult. There are several good solutions to help you squelch that sweet craving.

First, try the herb stevia in a cup of tea. Stevia does taste sweet, but it does not feed your yeast overgrowth. Research shows that it balances the body's blood sugar. You can adjust the amount of stevia according to your taste. (See our recipes in Part VII for more ways to use this valuable herb.) Artificial sweeteners are not on The Diet. They suppress the immune system.

Other ways to combat your sweet tooth are sprinkling apple cider vinegar on your vegetables, drinking it in water, and eating lots of cultured vegetables and young coconut water kefir. Besides providing an abundance of friendly bacteria, these enzyme-rich, high-quality, alkaline, expansive foods balance out the more contracting animal proteins and salty foods that make you crave acid-forming sugars.

The Diet uses the sweet-tasting vegetables liberally: onions, carrots, and butternut and acorn squash.

Fruits are ideal foods to help open and relax a woman's body just before her monthly cleansing, but are limited until she restores her body ecology. Do drink more water with freshly squeezed lemon or lime juice (with stevia if you want).

The nutrient-rich, high-protein green algae formulas are reported to have a remarkable ability to reduce and then eliminate sugar cravings.

In your meal planning, remember to balance expanding foods with contracting ones, sweet with salt. For example, when you eat contracting, salty foods, such as meat or eggs, balance them with expanding foods, such as raw vegetables and salad, using the 80/20 rule. This balance is critical. If your body becomes too contracted, you will start craving sugar and be tempted to abandon The Diet so you can satisfy that sweet taste. DON'T DO IT! Bring your body back into balance, and then eat along the middle of the Expansion/Contraction Continuum.

Kefir from milk added to The Diet as a breakfast food curbs cravings. Cleansing the colon does, too. A glass of water often stops any craving for sugar. Most of the time we are not hungry, but simply dehydrated.

Binges

It takes courage and willpower to stay on The Diet. One of the best ways to cultivate this is to hold a vision of yourself without any symptoms of candidiasis, a healed body and soul. Imagine what your life will be like, free from pain, free from all the symptoms that have stopped you from doing what you want to do in life. It's a feeling that you may not have had for a long time, but it can be recaptured; you can create it for yourself. Take encouragement from this book and from the many people who have used The Diet and healed themselves.

Sometimes, however, the urge to have some "forbidden" food is just overwhelming, and people eat a little—or a lot. If that happens to you, just go back on The Diet as soon as possible. Try not to wallow in self-criticism. Just resolve not to do that again, and know that The Diet ultimately will make you feel better and more balanced, so you will not have those cravings.

Our Antidote to a Sugar Binge

We often find that when people do slip off the Diet, drinking a six-ounce glass of water to which one tablespoon of apple cider vinegar has been added and/or eating 1/2 cup or more of the raw cultured vegetables or young coconut kefir as soon as possible reduces some of the usual negative symptoms. These alkaline-rich, cultured foods aid in digestion and convert sugars to useful lactic and acetic acid. They also supply living microorganisms that help keep the yeast under control.

Alcoholism and Bulimia

The Body Ecology Diet is especially healing for alcoholics. Alcoholics have candidiasis, and it has often spread to the liver. If they try to give up alcohol without understanding how to cope with the enormously powerful cravings of yeast organisms and a sugar addiction, they won't succeed. By following the Body Ecology Diet, with its elimination of sugars; consuming the herb stevia, raw cultured vegetables, apple cider vinegar, and probiotics; and eating in a balanced way (using the expansion/contraction principle), they have a much better chance. **Drinking two cups of young coconut kefir each day is remarkable for preventing cravings for sugar and alcohol**. Of course, an alcoholic still needs support on spiritual and emotional levels, too, but The Diet is critical.

People with bulimia also have a sugar addiction and a body-ecology imbalance. Bulimia is *not* only a self-image or emotional problem. Break the sugar addiction, conquer the yeast, restore the inner ecosystem, and while they are in counseling (learning how to feel better about themselves), watch anyone with an eating disorder become well . . . step by step.

If you find yourself craving sweets, try the following before giving in to the demands of the yeast:

- Drink several glasses of water close together; you may be dehydrated.

- Drink a cup of tea or a beverage with stevia.

- Eat 1/2 cup raw cultured vegetables or a glass of young coconut water kefir.

- Eat a leafy green salad with B.E.D. dressing.

- Sprinkle apple cider vinegar on lightly steamed vegetables.

Decide if the cause of your craving for sugar is:
- Your body attempting a contraction/expansion balance (are you eating foods that are too salty?)

- Yeast demanding to be fed

- Simple dehydration

The Woman/Sugar Hormone Connection

Women have a particularly difficult time with sugar cravings just before their monthly cleansing. Most unknowingly allow their bodies to become too contracted by eating too many contracting foods (salt and animal protein) or from too much stress just before this monthly event. They crave sugars as their bodies attempt to "open" or relax enough to shed the lining of the uterus. Furthermore, production of the hormone progesterone increases (as it should), causing an increase in the blood sugar. The yeast feed off this increased sugar, multiply, and demand more sugar-rich foods. Sugar depletes the adrenals . . . two magnificent organs that help produce progesterone. It harms the thyroid that regulates estrogen-progesterone balance. A progesterone deficiency takes place, and PMS symptoms (irritability, depression, tender breasts, puffiness) flare up. Vaginitis also occurs.

Obviously, if a woman is going to ever feel well, she must break the sugar habit. Thankfully, stevia added to your diet will safely satisfy your cravings yet will not cause a flare-up of your yeast infection.

Trusting Your Intuition

Can you trust your intuition about what your body needs to eat? If you drank breast milk as your first food; then graduated to vegetables, fruits, and grains; properly combined your foods; and ate lots of cultured foods, the answer would be yes. But with a body-ecology imbalance, you can never trust your intuition to tell you what your body needs. Billions of yeast and other unwelcome visitors living inside you are sending messages about what *they* want to eat (always a form of sugar). They do not care in the least about the needs of the body they live in.[17]

If you find yourself craving the healthy foods on the B.E.D., yes, listen to your body. For example, if you crave chicken, fish, or eggs, your body wants protein and/or has a need for more contracting and strengthening foods. The yeast are not asking, your body is.

Even if you are normally a vegetarian, at least eat some eggs. Food can be used as medicine to restore balance as needed. Once the balance is achieved, you will lose your taste for them again.

Once you've restored your body ecology, you can ask yourself before each meal, "What do I need?"

◦℘

Notes

[17] To better understand the spiritual cause behind our current physical condition, we should reflect on how very much like the yeast we are. We, in a similar fashion, have been living upon the earth, not caring or realizing that it has its needs, too. Like the yeast, we have been demanding what we want . . . and taking it. We've become a world of weak, sensitive, vulnerable bodies, mirroring the vulnerability of our planet.

Chapter 17

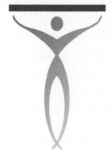

Traveling, Eating Out, and Snacking on the Body Ecology Diet

Travel

Travel, especially on airplanes, has a contracting, acid-forming impact on the body. Many people find that when their routines are changed by being in different time zones or just being away from home, their bodies react with symptoms of contraction and acidity, such as constipation, fatigue, headaches, or stomach upset. That's why people crave expansive foods like alcohol and sweets when they travel; their bodies are trying to get back into balance. Here's how to do it the right way.

Eat expansive, alkaline-forming foods. Fruits would be ideal, but since they are not on the B.E.D., the next best foods are raw vegetable juices, raw vegetables, then cooked vegetables, then grains. Avoid contracting foods such as animal protein and salt.

It's important to eat lightly, too. The digestive tract slows down when we travel, so lighter foods are easier to digest.

Drink lots of fluids—even more than usual. Put lemon or lime slices and a bit of stevia (if you have it) into water, preferably purified or mineral water. Drink fresh vegetable juices if you can find them (or bring some along on your trip).

For the most part, it's difficult to eat airline meals and stay on The Diet. Even the "vegetarian" meals that some airlines offer are poorly combined, poorly cooked, and made from frozen food, which has lost its "Ki" or life force. You might want to bring your own food.

Better yet, encourage the airlines to start offering fresh fruit and vegetable platters and light grain dishes. They could save a lot of money and contribute to their passengers' health. Or open an airport concession where you sell freshly squeezed vegetable and fruit juices for people to take on the plane!

Restaurants

No, it's not impossible to enjoy a restaurant meal while you are on The Diet. It just takes a little planning and a lot of will-power (or "won't" power, as in "I won't eat that"). Restaurants are used to requests that deviate from the menu. Many people have medical conditions or allergies that require special food, so you won't be alone in asking for what you want and what will support your health.

You can always get a delicious piece of fresh fish or grilled chicken breast with steamed veggies and a salad in any good restaurant. Order a plain salad with some lemon wedges to squeeze on top. Good restaurants have extra-virgin olive oil. Many people on the Body Ecology Diet carry with them a "salad dressing kit." They tuck a small travel pouch containing leak-proof plastic bottles filled with olive or roasted pumpkin seed oil, apple cider vinegar, and Herbamare or sea salt into their purse or briefcase. A pillbox filled with enzymes is great, too. I (Donna) also add a bottle of Body Ecology's stevia liquid concentrate to my kit.

Many restaurants list vegetables as side dishes. You might order two such dishes, like steamed broccoli and green beans. A tiny vial of Herbamare seasoning in your salad kit adds flavor to any steamed vegetable. Sometimes you will find an appetizer of a platter of raw veggies and a dip; just order it without the dip and ask for lemon wedges instead.

Restaurants sometimes serve small red skin potatoes with their entrees; try ordering them separately. You could combine them with a salad and/or a vegetable side dish for a perfect Body Ecology Diet meal. Because ghee does not require refrigeration, a small jar of ghee in that kit comes in very handy if the potatoes need seasoning.

Just make up your mind before you leave your house that you won't have bread, dessert, or a poorly combined meal when you dine out. Concentrate on enjoying the surroundings and the people you're with. If everyone at your table orders a cocktail before dinner, you order sparkling water with lemon or lime slices. Slip out that little dropper bottle of stevia liquid concentrate from your salad kit, and you won't feel like you're missing a thing.

People living in Atlanta are lucky, thanks to the R. Thomas Deluxe Grill on Peachtree Street. It offers wonderful Body Ecology–approved meals along with a regular menu of burgers.

Parties

Parties may be a bit more difficult because the range of food choices is narrower. A good trick is to eat either a full or partial meal at home before the party so you won't be tempted to eat "forbidden" foods once you're there. If you feel comfortable enough to bring a B.E.D. dish to share with others, most hosts and hostesses will appreciate your thoughtfulness— you might be surprised at others' interest in your new way of eating. Health is a popular topic of conversation everywhere these days.

Because your digestion is becoming more and more efficient and you have less of that bloated or full feeling after meals, you may feel hungry more often yet not want to eat a full meal. Here are some tips for good, quick snacks:

- Keep a bowl of celery and carrot sticks in the refrigerator.
- Use the Body Ecology Diet Salad Dressing as a "dip" for these and other cut-up fresh veggies.
- Eat baked blue corn chips with cultured vegetables.
- Munch on popcorn and carrot sticks.
- Try raw pumpkin seeds with celery sticks.

- Sip a glass of young coconut water kefir. (Great at bedtime.)

- Keep a pot of soup in the refrigerator so you can heat up a little bit of it at a time.

- Chew on some nori, the ocean vegetable used for wrapping sushi rolls. Dulse is good, too.

- Eat some young coconut meat or fermented kefir cheese.

- Cultured veggies mixed with young coconut kefir cheese are delicious. Roll this mixture up in a romaine lettuce leaf and enjoy.

As time passes, you'll figure out your own best ways to stay on The Diet. You'll invent ways to eat and recipes and ideas you can pass on to others. Feel free to send them to us as well; we'd love to hear from you. (See end of book for our e-mail address.)

❧

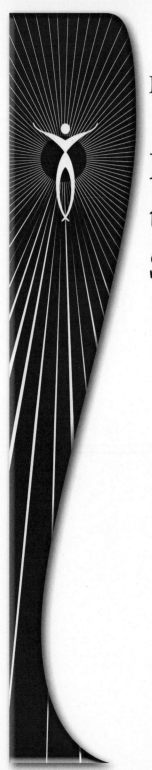

PART IV

Rebuilding
the Immune
System

Chapter 18

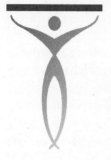

How to Care for Your Colon

For many people, bringing up the subject of colon hydrotherapy, or even *reading* this chapter, may be embarrassing, and your first inclination might be to avoid the topic altogether. But colon care and cleansing are critical to healing and knowing how to keep your body healthy.

When we say that it's essential to have a clean colon, we mean one free of toxins, waste material, and unhealthy microorganisms that accumulate in the waste material and on the walls, preventing the food you eat from being properly absorbed by your body. Many people have seven to ten pounds of old fecal matter in their colons, plus inches of hardened material on the walls of their small intestine, even if they have a bowel movement every day. When this accumulation is removed by various colon-cleansing procedures, the body is free to absorb the essential vitamins and minerals of the Body Ecology Diet, and accelerated healing begins.

Disease originates in the intestines, but health starts there as well. When waste cannot be properly eliminated, it accumulates in the colon and then backs up into the rest of the digestive tract, then the liver and kidneys. This causes unpleasant symptoms everywhere in the body. This can mean constipation, headaches, weight gain, skin problems, muscle and joint pain, depression, premature aging, and serious illnesses, including cancers. Even chronic diarrhea is a symptom of congestion somewhere in the intestines.

The digestive system (which includes the colon) is similar to the root system of a tree. A tree takes its nourishment and water through its root system, feeding them along the branches and out to the leaves. We take ours through the digestive tract, where the nutrients from food are carried into the bloodstream, then passed along to the various organs and absorbed into the cells of the body. In either system, if there is a blockage, or if poor-quality nutrients are taken in and distributed, the entire tree—or body—is thrown out of balance, and its very life is in danger.

What the Colon Does

The diagram on the right compares the length of the digestive tract to the average height of a human being. With such a long distance for food to travel, you can see the potential for blockages.

The colon is not merely a long tube used for waste elimination. Its most important function is to send water and essential vitamins and minerals from food into the body through the colon walls. But if the walls are blocked, those nutrients never reach their destination, and toxins are absorbed into the body. Gray hair comes from improper protein and mineral absorption. If adults had colons as pure and clean as an infant's, their hair would have rich, beautiful color!

The accumulation of waste on the walls of the colon provides the perfect breeding ground for parasites, yeast, and viruses. Many of us harbor viruses that only emerge when our immunity is low, and then we get flu or cold symptoms. The accumulation of toxins physically impairs elimination of feces and also can prevent friendly bacteria from colonizing and doing their work. It can become just like an oil spill: the environment is so polluted that even healthy animals and birds cannot survive.

Why Cleanse?

The way most of us eat these days, toxins do accumulate in our bodies, and they start in the digestive tract and colon. Fecal material can build up over the years, stretching the colon out of its proper shape and position within the body.

Even if you think you're in reasonably good health, if you're an adult, your digestive tract and colon undoubtedly have been abused and will profit from cleansing. If you do have a health problem, your digestive tract unquestionably is in poor condition. An initial, deliberate cleansing program and then restoring a robust inner ecosystem are essential to healing and staying young. If you start eating properly but don't cleanse the colon, you will slow down the healing process significantly. The two must go hand in hand.

We recognize the importance of cleaning our houses, or taking our cars in for regular maintenance to prolong their effectiveness—why not take care of our bodies just as well or better? The results will be even more rewarding: a long, vital life and excellent health. The colon is the most important place to start. If you begin by cleansing the colon, the other organs then automatically begin to eliminate their waste into it, as your body was designed to do. In this manner, the toxins and waste the body has stored—sometimes for years and years—can exit naturally.

Benefits of a Healthy Colon

Reestablishing the vitality of your colon is a key component of the Body Ecology way of life. It's just as important as eating the right foods. And once you've started the process, it becomes easier to stay on The Diet. As you accomplish this important goal, here are the results you can expect.

You will have much greater energy and vigor and, at the same time, an inner calm and improved mental clarity. You will sleep better. You will be less likely to crave sugar; your body will be better able to absorb nutrients; and you'll soon be able to taste the sweetness in foods such as onions, carrots, and fruits. You will certainly look brighter, and your muscles and skin will be well hydrated. Bloating will be reduced, and you will maintain a healthier weight.

A healthy colon greatly slows the aging process. When the body absorbs vitamins and minerals properly, the signs of age, such as gray hair and wrinkles, will be slower to appear.

Finally, a properly functioning colon reduces the need for strong cleansings; you will have gentler cleansings that you don't even notice.

What Others Say about Colon Cleansing

"The road to health is the one that begins with an understanding and commitment to cleanse and detoxify the body, to restore balance, peace and harmony. . . ."
—*Bernard Jensen, D.C., Ph.D.*

"Colon health emphasizes prevention rather than cure. It is the most important step in maintaining or regaining vital health. If the sewer system in your home is backed up, your entire home is affected. Should it be any different with your body?"
—*Norman Walker, D.Sc., health expert who died at the age of 109*

The Secret to Longevity

Cleansing is not only a basic principle of the Body Ecology Diet, it is an essential life goal. It is the secret to a long life, to looking fabulous and staying disease free. Faithful attention to cleansing will prevent diseases that we often assume come naturally with old age. These diseases represent the accumulation of a lifetime of toxins and impurities that the body has never cleaned out.

Remember, babies are born with super-clean digestive tracts. They build a strong immune system with friendly bacteria promoted by mother's milk. When they eat properly, they do not store toxins in their digestive tracts and quickly eliminate waste matter. If we could maintain our digestive tracts and colons in the condition of a healthy year-old child, our life expectancy would be much higher than it is now, and we would be free of many of the diseases affecting us in our old age.

How Foods We Eat Move Through the Colon

Putrefaction is the process by which foods decay within the colon and generate toxins and a foul odor. Ideally, the colon should be clean enough that foods spend minimal time passing through it and do not putrefy. Much of this depends on what foods are eaten and the actions of the friendly microflora that make up your inner ecosystem.

Transit time is the time it takes from eating food until its residues are expelled from the body. The average transit time in Western civilization is 65 to 100 hours![18] Once the colon has been cleansed and a healthy diet is maintained, that time can be reduced to 18 to 24 hours.

The ideal, healthy stool is neither runny nor mushy; it drops from the body within seconds after one sits on the toilet; it is fully formed, but crumbles into little pieces when the toilet is flushed; and it is free from the clay-like appearance that comes from mucus-forming foods.

What Damages Your Intestines?

Sugar, flour products, and unfermented dairy products are among the most damaging foods to the colon. Poor food combining is damaging as well. For example, eating a meal that contains a protein (like turkey) and a sugar (like in pumpkin pie) is harmful. These are all very mucus-forming; the mucus slowly accumulates on the walls of your intestines, and even if you are now eating the healthiest, most mineral- or vitamin-rich foods available, the mucus barrier will prevent those nutrients from being absorbed through the intestinal walls and into the cells in your body.

When poorly digested, animal foods (meat, fish, eggs, poultry) produce dangerous by-products and toxins that create inflammation. Disorders ranging from diverticulitis to cancer can result.

When you lack an inner ecosystem teeming with beneficial bacteria, **improperly prepared grains** will be poorly digested and cause gas, bloating, and inflammation. Millions of people are now gluten intolerant and one reason is that their intestines lack the "grain-loving" microflora that can digest gluten. Body Ecology's Whole Grains Biotic, a gluten-free beverage made from a wonderful variety of whole grains that are fermented with bacteria and good yeast, can help solve this problem (see Shopping List or website for more information).

Overeating also damages the colon. It's imperative to eat only until you're about 80 percent full to give your digestive tract a chance to function properly. Once that food is absorbed and on its way through the system, if you're hungry again, go ahead and eat more. Some people eat several small meals throughout the day and never gain weight (as long as they food-combine properly[19]) because their bodies are absorbing and eliminating correctly. Weight gain results when the intestines accumulate toxins and when food is poorly digested. Create a healthy digestive tract with clean intestines and you'll find it easy to maintain your ideal weight.

Stress and anger—the high-impact forces in our daily lives—cause the body to become contracted and uptight; this delays or stops elimination, and constipation results.

Fatigue—not enough sleep or rest—means we don't have the energy to eliminate. The bowel movement is a cleansing, and cleansing requires energy. Some people find they can relieve constipation just by getting more sleep.

Ways to Cleanse Your Colon

Many excellent books go into more detail than we can here about methods of cleansing the colon (see the Bibliography). However, here are various therapies you might try:

Enemas

People have used enemas since ancient times to aid healing. In fact, until about 70 years ago, medical doctors frequently prescribed them as part of a normal cure for disease, saving many lives. Doctors would often make home visits and prescribe an enema to bring down a fever. Now, medical professionals have little or no training in the value of enemas for helping the body quickly eliminate waste. There are two types of enemas: cleansing and retention. Coffee enemas (used to open the bile duct so toxins can be released from the liver) are *retention* enemas. The *cleansing* enemas are not retained or held in the body for long; they are used to rinse out the colon. Use filtered water in an enema bag . . . or better yet, an enema bucket . . . found at most hospital supply stores. With an enema, it is easy to add minerals, tinctures, and herbal teas to the water; and this can be very therapeutic. (Do a quick search on the Internet for more information on different types of enemas and how to administer them.)

Colonics

Colonic irrigation offers a pleasant and convenient way to hydrate and cleanse. In addition, it bathes the entire length of the colon using about ten gallons of water per session. (In contrast, an enema only uses two quarts of water.) When administered properly, colonics are safe, painless, and clean. Find a therapist you feel comfortable with, who has been trained to fill the colon very slowly with filtered water and who uses disposable tubing and attachments. The colon therapist should remain with you at all times during your session. After each colonic a cup or two of water and other nutritional substances such as minerals, wheat grass, vitamin C, and B vitamins can be implanted directly into the colon to provide nourishment to your entire body. Unless they have a prescription from your doctor to do an implant, colon therapists are not allowed to administer them. This is something you can do yourself at home.

Colon cleansing will also help cleanse your liver and your lymph system. It's essential to use purified water, water without chlorine or other matter, since chlorine kills friendly bacteria. Once your colon is free of blockages, re-toned and well hydrated again, colonics and enemas can be used whenever you are ill or are "cleansing." Contrary to popular belief, colon cleansing will not wash away the beneficial microflora since they are safely nestled into the mucosal lining. Colonics do wash out friendly bacteria contained in the stool if there are any, but a toxic colon doesn't have friendly bacteria anyway. In the early stage of cleansing, eliminating yeast, parasites, and blocks of fecal material is important so that friendly bacteria will be able to colonize inside you.

After the colon is cleansed, you'll want to colonize your colon by taking probiotics orally, by colonic implants*, and by eating raw cultured vegetables and drinking kefir made with milk or from young coconut water.

TIP: After a colonic, you may feel tired. Go home and rest, putting on warm, comfortable clothing. Pamper yourself. Take a warm bath and go to bed early. Eat light, easy-to-digest foods such as Vitality SuperGreen drink, vitality broth, steamed vegetables, and/or one of the B.E.D. pureed soups. Avoid raw vegetables. Sip on water with added minerals or potassium-rich apple cider vinegar. It will restore electrolytes that are briefly lost when the stool is cleansed from the colonic.**

* Our favorite implant after cleaning your colon: 1 cup young coconut kefir, 2 capsules of Body Ecology's Ancient Earth Minerals (open capsules and dissolve), and 2 capsules of vitamin C or 1/2 tsp. vitamin C powder.

** Into 4 cups of water, add: 2 cups red potato peelings (cut 1/2″ thick); 2 cups celery stalks (chopped); 2 cups celery tops; 1 carrot (chopped); 1 small onion (chopped). Simmer, covered, for 30 minutes; strain liquid; and drink 8 oz. every 2–3 hours.

Herbs

Some herbs, such as aloe, senna, and cascara, act as laxatives. They are okay to use occasionally when you are very constipated, but only for a very short time. They weaken the adrenals. Weak adrenals mean weak energy. It takes energy to produce a healthy stool. Weak adrenals, an underactive thyroid, a congested liver, and low stomach acid are four common causes of constipation.

Psyllium vs. Flax Seed

Colon cleansing products often contain psyllium or bentonite, substances that virtually pull impacted waste material off the colon walls. When using psyllium, **it's crucial to drink a lot of water**. Psyllium is a bulking agent and will actually cause constipation unless you wash it through with enough liquid—certainly eight glasses of water a day. We prefer more gentle products such as ground flax fiber (found in Vitality SuperGreen). Genesis Today has an excellent fiber blend called 4Fiber with organic flaxseed, noni fiber, and wonderful herbs. (See Shopping List.) Research on flax fiber shows that it protects your colon from cancer and is antiviral, antibacterial, and antifungal. The B.E.D. grain-like seeds, soaked and cooked with more water porridge-style, also provide excellent stimulation to the intestines, helping to create a healthy stool.

Foods That Assist Colon Cleansing

- Garlic is well known for its medicinal and cleansing value. It has antifungal, antimicrobial properties and can relieve gas, bloating, and water retention; it also helps digestion. You can swallow small cloves of garlic whole. Cook with it as much as possible; many of our recipes include garlic. It also comes in various supplements from which the odor has been removed.

- Foods high in fiber, such as grains and vegetables, also enhance cleansing. Fruits are high in fiber and water content—excellent for cleansing—but unfortunately many are not on The Diet, at least at first. Sour fruits are tolerated right from the start, and you may be able to add more fruits soon if you are eating fermented foods. Green smoothies made from raw vegetables and chlorophyll-rich foods, such as leafy greens, provide the fiber that friendly bacteria love. Cultured vegetables are excellent high-fiber foods.

- Eating a salad with the Body Ecology Diet Salad Dressing each day will provide you with good fiber. The apple cider vinegar in the dressing is especially healing; it will help reestablish those colonies of friendly bacteria once the colon has been cleaned.

- Foods on The Diet that accelerate cleansing include green smoothies and raw vegetable juices (with added fiber) taken on an empty stomach, daikon, green onions, leeks, chives, turnips, spaghetti squash, fenugreek, and curry powder.

- Fermented foods (see Chapter 14) help keep the colon clean and allow friendly bacteria to grow.

- Flax seed tea is excellent for healing the colon. It's especially valuable if you suffer from leaky gut or irritable bowel syndrome, a spastic colon, colitis, or bloody stools. To make: Pour 12 ounces of boiling water over a tablespoon of flax seed and steep for 30 minutes or longer. (Overnight is even better.) Drain and drink the liquid. You can also use chia seeds if you prefer.

Understanding Intestinal Bacteria

In general, there are three types of bacteria in the digestive tract: pathogenic (hostile), beneficial (friendly), and neutral. Microbiologists don't have the final answers on what all the bacteria do; some colonize and some are transient, but even the transient ones can be helpful. The beneficial bacteria are easily disturbed, and especially affected by stress. The pathogens attach themselves to tissues and develop sites of infection.

It is estimated that more than 1,000 species of bacteria inhabit our digestive tracts, weighing up to three and a half pounds! It could take a year or more to accomplish a complete bacteriological analysis of one tiny sample of human feces.[20] This indicates the complexity of our inner ecosystems, and shows why it is important to be aware of different factors— such as antibiotics, birth-control pills, or a high-sugar diet— that can upset the inner balance.

The type of food we eat directly influences the type of friendly bacteria that proliferate within our systems. A diet rich in meat and fat produces different bacteria than a high-complex-carbohydrate/lacto-vegetarian diet. All friendly bacteria, however, produce enzymes that aid digestion. A high concentration of friendly bacteria greatly improves transit time and also plays a vital role in breaking up waste that has accumulated on the colon walls.

Given the key role of friendly bacteria in our ecosystems, it is important to continually replenish them with probiotics and probiotic foods.

How Do You Know When Your Colon Is Better?

First, you'll feel better—maybe better than you have in years. Gas, bloating, and many of your other chronic symptoms will disappear. You should have more energy and simply feel happier. Your breath will be fresh. If you can wake up in the morning without bad breath and without having to brush your teeth, that's a good barometer that your digestive tract is in good shape.

Parasites

Many people believe that parasites exist only in those who are exposed to unsanitary living conditions. This is not so. Millions of Americans have them in one form or another.[21]

Parasites are common in the digestive tract of everyone. Their eggs and larvae are on the foods we eat, and we infect ourselves when we touch objects with our hands and put our hands in our mouths. Many of them are relatively harmless and live, breed, and die inside us. Most of them are microscopic. Pathogenic bacteria parasites, like giardia, *Blastocystis hominis*, and *Clostridia difficile,* cause serious infections and gut dysbiosis. *Candida albicans*, a fungus, is also an intestinal parasite. When we lack a hardy inner ecosystem, we are more susceptible to parasite infections. Parasites can attack anyone who is in a weakened state. For instance, parasites are frequently present in people who have nutritional and/or immune deficiencies. The symptoms caused by parasites can mimic those of other diseases, such as flu or Candida Related Complex (CRC), and parasites can even exist without causing any symptoms at all. The first three parasite infections mentioned above must usually be treated with an antibiotic before you can reestablish a healthy inner ecosystem in your intestines. Stay on the Body Ecology Diet when you use an antibiotic, and continue to eat and drink probiotic foods. Plantarum, the bacteria in our cultured vegetable starter, is especially resistant to antibiotics and will not be destroyed. Antibiotics and fermented foods should be taken two hours apart.

Parasites are difficult to diagnose. If you think your candida is under control, but you still have symptoms such as gas, bloating, and allergic reactions to foods that do not feed yeast, there's a good possibility that other types of parasites may be the culprit. There are various stool tests that your doctor can order for you to confirm a diagnosis and type of parasite.

However, since so many people do have undetected parasites, it can't hurt to go through a program of parasite control periodically. Swallowing a whole clove of garlic is effective against parasites. Health-food stores have various preparations you might want to try. We, of course, recommend Body Ecology's EcoClear™.

Other Aspects of Colon Care

- Massage helps to reduce stress and relax the body, making elimination easier.

- Acupuncture can help stimulate the large intestine and balance it in relation to other organs.

- Drinking enough water—eight glasses a day—is essential to proper functioning of the digestive tract and relief of constipation.

- Breathing deeply has a very beneficial effect on the large intestine. In Oriental medicine, the lungs and large intestine have a very strong relationship. So anything you do to strengthen the lungs also strengthens the large intestine. When you take deep breaths, you can actually feel your abdomen relax. People who smoke have weak large intestines.

- Exercise, of course, helps all areas of the body and especially the large intestine and lungs. A 30-minute walk each day can be the most effective exercise for improving elimination. Bike riding is great, too. The thigh muscles are on the same meridian, or energy pathway, as the colon, so stimulating these muscles will help tone and relax the colon.

- A healthy colon ensures a healthy liver. Your liver eliminates its impurities by producing bile and then handing that toxic bile off to the gallbladder to store temporarily. When you eat a meal, the gallbladder drops this bile down into the small intestine. Once there, the bile digests the fats you ate and stimulates peristalsis so that the digested food moves down into your colon. If the colon is not eliminating as it should, those same toxins are reabsorbed back into the liver once again. A diet high in refined fats and oils, overeating, and drugs all damage the liver and can cause it to "back up" with toxins; this in turn can result in problems with the skin, eyes, and joints, especially the knees. So this is why many people with CRC also have skin problems: the colon is clogged, the liver is clogged, and waste tries to exit the body via the skin (see Chapter 21: The Liver). Body Ecology's LivAmend with New Zealand wasabi extract contains herbs that stimulate bile to flow from the liver so that toxins can leave smoothly.

How to Maintain and Nourish a Clean Colon

There are several more actions you can take to make sure your colon is functioning at its optimal level.

During the night while you sleep, your intestines become dehydrated. Right after you wake up, also wake up your intestine by sipping 12 to 16 ounces of warm or room-temperature, mineral water. Drinking and eating sour and fermented foods throughout the morning stimulates peristaltic movement in your intestines. A healthy colon will ideally eliminate in the morning and be ready to process new foods.

A daily bowel movement is desirable for adults, and there's nothing wrong with one after each meal. (Remember, babies, with their pristine digestive tracts, often move their bowels after each meal.) But ultimately how often we eliminate and how much we eliminate is determined by how much we eat and assimilate.

We've been conditioned to suppress the reflex that prompts the bowels to move each time the stomach fills up. We often wait until just the right time or place. But as part of a colon improvement program, it would be helpful to retrain your bowels. Some colon therapists recommend excusing yourself about ten minutes after a meal and sitting on the toilet, exercising the abdominal muscles and encouraging even the slightest urge to move the bowels.

Adding chlorophyll to your water helps maintain a good acid/alkaline balance and supports the recolonizing of friendly bacteria in your body ecology; it adds oxygen. You also encourage growth of friendly bacteria by consuming unsalted raw cultured vegetables; raw apple cider vinegar; young coconut and milk kefir; probiotic liquids, like Cocobiotic, InnergyBiotic, and dong quai; and, of course, probiotic supplements found in your health food-store.

Help from Probiotics

Into a blender add 1 cup of water, 1 teaspoon of a probiotic powder blend, 1 teaspoon of alcohol-free vanilla flavoring, 1 heaping teaspoon of lecithin granules (optional), and a few drops of our liquid stevia concentrate. Blend for a few seconds, and you have the Body Ecology Diet "acidophilus milk." You can drink it first thing in the morning on an empty stomach, waiting at least one half hour before eating food. It's great for your colon. If you use a dairy-free probiotic brand, you can also use it as "milk" on top of Arrowhead Mills puffed millet cereal. Add a pinch of cinnamon if you'd like.

You might consider colonic implants to give you added energy and enhance the color and texture of your skin. You can implant probiotics, minerals, and/or chlorophyll, separately or together. The best time is right after a colonic or home enema and right before bedtime.

Put at least 2 teaspoons of probiotics and/or 2 tablespoons of liquid chlorophyll with liquid minerals and 4 ounces of purified water or young coconut kefir into an enema bag or bucket. Insert it into your colon, and when you lie down to go to sleep, the colon will be able to retain this amount of liquid.

Fasting

In Chinese medicine, food is used to heal. Eating high-quality foods is the best path to cleansing and healing; people with immune-compromised conditions are usually too weak to fast. But as you get stronger and healthier and want to cleanse very deliberately, you might try a modified fast. Maybe one day a week or twice a month, drink and eat only the cultured foods on The Diet. Fasting gives the digestive tract a chance to rest.

Later in your healing, you can modify your pattern again, such as by drinking water and lemon juice throughout the day, and eating only a light vegetable meal in the afternoon. Once you are able to tolerate grapefruit, you can use it like lemons and lemon juice. A day when you drink only warm vegetable broth (called "pot liquor" in the South) makes an ideal modified fast.

You can also fast on milk kefir diluted with water for a day. The Russians and Turks do this all the time, and it is a famous cure in Russian health sanitariums.

Milk by nature is dehydrating, so adding water makes it more balanced and medicinal. In ancient Ayurvedic texts you will find this kefir/water mixture mentioned as a cure for many digestive problems. They refer to it as "curd water."

TIP: Fast only on days when you can also rest, such as the weekend, to give your body the full advantage of the cleansing process.

Pacing Your Cleansing

Toxins sometimes leave the body faster than the body can eliminate them through its usual systems, and this is when a cleansing reaction occurs. We've already mentioned this Herxheimer reaction, when you may have symptoms such as a flu-like soreness, skin eruptions, dizziness, itching, emotional upheaval, sleep disorders, or intensification of a pre-existing symptom. You do have some control over how smoothly and comfortably you cleanse. If you begin The Diet and combine it with a series of colonics or home enemas, you will avoid a buildup of too many toxins . . . more than your body can handle at one time.

Final reminders for maintaining a healthy colon: stay on the Body Ecology Diet, adding suitable foods as you can tolerate them; remember to follow the food-combining rules; and exercise. Cleansing and healing is a lifelong process. Honor the principle of step by step so you don't become discouraged.

The Deer Exercise

The deer exercise comes from the physical, mental, and spiritual teachings of Taoism, an ancient religion and way of life. It is so named because the deer continually stimulates its sexual glands by constantly contracting and relaxing its anal muscles and moving its tail from side to side. The inner energy this creates travels to the antlers, which are valued in Chinese medicine for their great healing powers.

In people, the exercise builds sexual desire, which is often weak in those with candidiasis. It has other important physical benefits, however.

Main Benefits

It tones the anal muscles and colon, aiding peristaltic action and reducing transit time. It prevents colitis. As we age, the muscles of the colon and the bladder tend to become loose and flaccid, and that is why many older people have a difficult time controlling these functions. Deterioration of the rectal and anal muscles can also hasten the onset of hemorrhoids and cancer; exercising them reverses this process.

In men, the deer exercise also strengthens the prostate and helps prevent disease, weakness, and enlargement or dysfunction of the prostate. In women, it stimulates the vaginal muscles, helping prevent and cure such problems as menstrual disorders, infections, and vaginitis.

How to Do It

The following description of the deer exercise comes from *The Book of Internal Exercises,* by Stephen T. Chang with Richard C. Miller (Strawberry Hill Press, San Francisco, Calif., 1978).

Do the exercise in the morning and evening. Sit in a comfortable position. Tighten the muscles around your anal opening as hard as you can, and hold this as long as you are comfortably able. (Women should tighten the vaginal muscles as well.) When done properly, this feels as if air is being drawn up into the rectum.

Don't force the process, but perform the exercise until you are tired. Stop, then repeat it when you are rested. At first, you may only be able to hold the sphincter muscles tight for several seconds. After a few weeks, if you persist, you will be able to hold them much longer without feeling tired or strained. If you do the exercise properly, you'll be aware of a pleasant feeling traveling from the base of the anus, through the spinal column, to the top of the head.

Notes

[18] Gray, 1986.

[19] If you eat frequently throughout the day, you can assist your food combining by devoting one day only to grains and/or starchy vegetables with land and ocean vegetables; another day, combine only protein with vegetables.

[20] Chaitow and Trenev, *Probiotics*, 1990.

[21] Luc De Schepper's *Peak Immunity* has a good discussion of possible symptoms and cures for parasites.

❧

Chapter 19

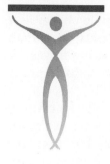

Special Information: Women, Men, Children

Each of us is unique; each of us has different needs and diverse paths to healing. However, we can generalize about different groups of people, based on our observations, and learn what will keep them healthy.

The Nature of Woman

According to the ancient principle of yin/yang (contraction/expansion), the essential nature of woman is yin and contractive. Water is often used as a symbol describing the true essence of woman. Water is fluid, flexible, yielding to resistance; yet it is persistent in getting to where it must go. It seeks a downward path representing humbleness (not submissiveness). When it is calm, it can be gentle and still, but it also has the power to become fierce, angry, and destructive. Indispensable to all, water's positive, accepting energy nurtures and brings forth life.

In contrast, man's nature is more like the energy of fire. Traditionally, man's role in society and the family has been more outward, expanding, forceful . . . arousing and inspiring . . . more fervent . . . conquering and intense.

It is well recognized that man has some female energy and woman has some male energy, but the essential natures of man and woman remain quite different. Both energies are necessary for creation, and a positive balance of the two allows many harmonious arrangements to take place.

Philosophers can have a wonderful time reflecting upon this yin/yang phenomenon, but for our purposes we want to understand how woman's nature influences her need for certain foods. What foods will give her the energy she needs to carry out her important role in her family and in society?

What Foods Are Best?

Foods that maintain the soft, fluid, accepting, yet powerful nature of a woman are *grains*, *vegetables*, and *fruit*. Salt and foods containing salt (including animal foods) cause contraction. Too much contraction hardens a woman's body, creating too much fire energy. Dairy products often have hormones that interfere with the delicate balance of a woman's own hormonal system. Sugar depletes a woman's body of essential minerals, those same minerals that determine her beauty and strength throughout her life and that during pregnancy help create new life.

Because of her receptive, intuitive qualities and her mission to bear new life, a woman's body tends to gather and store energy. As a protection for her and for her baby, nature gave her a body that processes food more efficiently and stores it away for future use. A woman, then, needs less food than a man, and when she eats too much, it is stored as fat. She also needs less animal protein. Too much and/or improperly digested protein causes dark, odorous, clotted, and stringy menstrual blood.

Sexual Organs Affected by Foods

A woman's sexual-organ system is very delicate and can be damaged by poor-quality food, excessive sugar, salt, and dairy foods. Dairy products not only contain hormones that interfere with the female hormones, but unfermented, pasteurized, and homogenized dairy is so mucus-forming that it is linked to serious disorders such as infertility from blocked fallopian tubes, cancer of the breast and cervix, endometriosis, menstrual cramps, heavy menstrual flow, tender breasts, ovarian tumors and cysts, and vaginal infections.

Sugar weakens and upsets a woman's delicate endocrine balance much more than it does a man's. In addition, especially around the time of her monthly period, too much salt can cause her body to become too contracted, which inhibits the shedding of the uterine lining.

Women and Candida

Dr. William Crook lists several reasons women develop yeast-connected health problems more than men or children:

- Hormonal changes connected with the normal menstrual cycle, as well as hormonal changes during pregnancy and adolescence, encourage yeast overgrowth.

- Birth-control pills can lead to candidiasis.

- Teenage girls, very concerned about their complexions, often start long-term acne treatment with antibiotics—and this promotes yeast overgrowth.

- The anatomy of the vagina provides an ideal place for candida colonization.

- The anatomy of the urethra leads women to experience more urinary-tract problems than men; antibiotics are often prescribed for this.

Caring for the Birth Canal (Vagina)

The birth canal is much more than an occasional passageway for birth; it continually functions as an avenue for cleansing. A channel to the outside, it permits unnecessary waste and damaging toxins to leave a woman's body. Constantly sloughing off toxins, it allows her body to stay cleaner and healthier . . . a protection for the children she might bear and a reason women outlive men. Women have more opportunities to cleanse.

A woman's emotional state is very much linked to the health of her sexual-organ system and to the condition of her birth canal: if the birth canal is irritated, diseased, or the pH out of balance, the woman will feel out of sorts. Once these conditions are corrected, she'll feel better.

Yeast infections can be localized in the birth canal, but today many women have developed *systemic* candidiasis: it occurs throughout the entire body. Since the body is designed to constantly rid itself of dangerous parasites, it will eliminate those yeast organisms (especially those colonized around the sexual organs) through the vagina. This creates much confusion for a woman. When she eats foods that feed the yeast, they will reproduce and cause damage to her system. Once she is on the Body Ecology Diet, they begin dying, millions of them leaving her body through her birth canal. Therefore, even though she is conquering her yeast problem, she could see signs of vaginal discharge for a very long time. It is important, then, for a woman to know how to care for this area until her body finishes cleansing itself of the yeast.

The environment of the vagina should be slightly acidic, and friendly bifidus bacteria only grow well in an acidic world. An alkaline condition encourages unfriendly bacteria to take hold, so it's important to maintain a clean, acidic vagina. (Male sperm is alkaline.)

Douche with apple cider vinegar and water to achieve an acidic condition. Traditional doctors might advise douching only once a month, after menstruation; this is fine once you are completely well. For now, it's perfectly safe to douche with apple cider vinegar once, twice, or more times a week, depending on your condition and especially after making love. Make sure it's raw, organic apple cider vinegar.

DOUCHE RECIPE: 1/4 cup raw, organic apple cider vinegar in 1 quart of distilled or purified water.

Following this cleansing, you can implant friendly bacteria into the birth canal by dissolving a probiotic powder (*Lactobacillus bifidus*) in a small amount of distilled water (2–4 oz.), then inserting it using the equivalent of a turkey baster—a small bulb or sack you can put the liquid in, with a way to squirt it into the vagina. (A travel douche bag works well, too.) This method works better than probiotic suppositories, because the liquid penetrates into the folds and crevices of the vaginal cavity, where the actual colonization takes place. The optimal time to do this is before bed, when you have the best chance of retaining that liquid. Remember, the goal is to have the friendly bacteria colonize in the vagina and grow on their own.

You can also add chlorophyll to the probiotic solution; chlorophyll provides oxygen for the friendly bacteria.

Tea tree oil is another excellent, gentle douche that is antifungal and antibacterial and leaves a fresh, clean feeling in the vagina. This essential oil comes from a tree that grows in Australia. It is available in health-food stores. Tea tree oil also comes in suppositories. You can obtain similar results by saturating a tampon with the oil and inserting it at bedtime.

Once you begin *eating* cultured veggies and the two kefirs, you'll soon notice a change in your vagina, too. Amazingly, cultured foods eaten by mouth soon start colonizing in the vagina. Starting our baby daughters on these cultured foods is very wise.

DOUCHE RECIPE: 1 teaspoon tea tree oil in 500 ml. (2 cups) distilled or purified water.

Making Love

A man's semen is alkaline, so after intercourse it is important to restore the acidic condition of the vagina. In addition, candida can be passed back and forth during sex, so the woman can protect herself by douching, then implanting with friendly bacteria. If you do this regularly, in addition to taking other steps to heal yourself, this act of personal care will have a beneficial effect.

Candida and Sex Drive

A woman's sex drive can easily wane if she has an overgrowth of candida. In a sort of vicious cycle, she doesn't feel well, she becomes hard to live with, she has physical symptoms that are not conducive to love-making—and then her relationship can be affected. It's very important to use the physical connection of intercourse as a way of keeping a relationship healthy.

In ancient times, Oriental healers viewed love-making as an art form and believed it had the power to restore well-being. Since woman's nature is to receive and accumulate energy, making love and releasing this stored energy through orgasm rebalances a woman and helps her feel much happier:

more relaxed, accepting, intuitive, giving, and nurturing. The energy of intercourse used in a pure and honorable way can be a spiritual, emotional, and physical aid to healing.

It's a wonder that Wendy K.'s marriage held together at all. It started out like a fairy tale: she fell in love in college, married her sweetheart Eric when they graduated, and two years later stopped taking birth-control pills so they could have their first child. But it was not an easy pregnancy, and she didn't feel much like having sex even during the early months. After the baby was born, she went back on birth-control pills. But the demands of motherhood and a career kept her hopping, and she was often too busy or tired to relax and enjoy sex with Eric.

When their son was three years old, the burden eased. They started to enjoy each other again and decided to have another baby. It was another difficult pregnancy, with frequent indigestion, vaginitis, headaches, fatigue, and irritability. Their daughter was born two months premature, creating a strain on Wendy and Eric's nerves and finances.

With two young children in the house, Eric working long hours to advance his career, and Wendy trying to work part-time, they hardly had a moment to themselves. Wendy had frequent vaginal itching and discharges, rectal itching, headaches, and muscle pains. She was a good mother but didn't take very good care of herself, always eating on the run and never allocating time to an exercise program for herself. She was tired and had absolutely no interest in sex.

At first Eric was very understanding, but after a while he started losing patience and wanted to know what happened to that loving, alluring college sweetheart he'd married. Wendy and Eric started fighting more and more.

Finally, they went to a counselor, who gave them some advice that helped add balance to their marriage. This counselor also happened to know about CRC and the Body Ecology Diet and recommended that both Wendy and Eric try The Diet. They did, and Wendy immediately began to feel better and have more energy. Her vaginitis cleared up, and her nerves calmed down. She and Eric were able to spend more quality time together and put joy and sex back into their marriage.

Pregnancy

During pregnancy, a woman's hormonal balance changes dramatically. If her body ecology is weak and she lacks adequate friendly bacteria, this leads to a condition of yeast overgrowth.

More and more babies are being delivered by Caesarean section, and their mothers are given antibiotics to prevent infection. These antibiotics kill any friendly bacteria a mother may have in her system, and they can be passed on to the baby in breast milk, causing trouble for the baby's immature ecosystem. Babies can easily develop infections when they have no internal body ecology and only fragile immune systems to protect them from unfriendly bacteria and viruses.

Throughout pregnancy, and especially if a mother-to-be must take antibiotics, the Body Ecology Diet is critical. Its total exclusion of foods that feed the yeast and its large amounts of cultured vegetables and probiotics (especially *Bifidus infantis*) will help her immensely. Still, she should not be discouraged if her yeast condition does not subside. The high amount of progesterone in her blood increases the amount of sugar, and the yeast will thrive even though she is not feeding them.

The good news is that childbirth is one of the best times to conquer this condition permanently—if you follow The Diet strictly and eliminate all forms of sugars. The act of giving birth is part of the wondrous arrangement of cleansing. The afterbirth and bloody materials that are sloughed off immediately after the baby is born, and the bloody discharge that follows for several weeks, provide a vehicle for yeast and toxins to leave the body.

The sudden hormonal changes that take place and the presence of healing agents that are designed to repair any damage from the birth give the new mother an opportunity to become even stronger than she was before her pregnancy. If she takes large amounts of the right probiotics, eats very, very well for four to six weeks after the baby is born, and rests to the point of doing nothing except caring for the precious new life given to her, a woman can emerge from the demanding process of pregnancy with an almost new body. (Please reread the chapters on cultured vegetables, young coconut kefir and kefir cheese, and kefir from milk. They contain important information for pregnant and nursing mothers.)

A Word of Caution

It's especially important for a pregnant woman to maintain a healthy vagina so that candida will not transfer to the baby as it passes through the birth canal. Check with your doctor first, but we have found that douching with probiotics, apple cider vinegar, and tea tree oil is fine during pregnancy. Discontinue just before you think your cervix will start to dilate.

About the Colon

Even before a woman becomes pregnant, she should work to create a clean, properly functioning colon. The high levels of progesterone in a pregnant woman drastically slow transit time of food and waste as they pass through the digestive tract; that's why pregnant women so often are constipated. The slower transit allows more time for the mother and the baby to absorb nutrients from the food, but if there is excess waste material built up in the colon, that absorption will be impeded. In fact, toxins will be absorbed, not vitamins and minerals. (See Chapter 18 to learn how to improve the health of your digestive system.)

Monthly Cycle

Remember, menstruation is a cleansing, and women should consider it a wonderful opportunity to eliminate toxins and become even healthier. Let's review the steps that make it easy to appreciate this monthly miracle.

- After you ovulate, reduce the amount of salt and contracting foods (especially animal proteins) you take in, so the body will not retain fluids and will easily let go of the uterine lining.

- Maintain this through the end of your period. Afterward, you can slightly increase your salt intake, perhaps by eating more contracting foods than you otherwise might (although still balancing them with expanding foods).

- Get plenty of rest during your period. Plan quiet activities. Cleansing takes energy. Estrogen and progesterone levels are low now, so you won't have a lot of energy.

- Eat well. Do not overeat, and do not stray from The Diet or binge on foods with sugar, which could wreak havoc in your system.

- All-alkaline meals (especially green vegetable juices and vegetable soups) are great when your period begins.

Once a woman knows she has a candida overgrowth and knows what to do about it, she can get well, with her own determination and help from the Body Ecology Diet.

Men and Candida

The damp, moldy, fungal nature of yeast dampens the fire nature of man. Candidiasis, while it is not as common as among women, is weakening many men in America today and has become a serious threat to the well-being of the family unit and to society.

Men are traditionally less likely to go to the doctor if they don't feel well and, therefore, are less likely to have taken antibiotics. They also don't have the contributing factors of monthly hormonal changes, birth-control pills, and multiple pregnancies. Nevertheless, candidiasis does strike men and is always present in people with cancer and with AIDS.

For the most part, candida affects different organs in a man than in a woman. In women, the yeast overgrowth often first manifests in the hormonal system, sexual organs, and the digestive tract, surfacing as vaginitis, PMS, constipation, gas, bloating, acne, and fatigue. In men, the yeast usually colonize first in the digestive tract and cause digestive disorders. As the condition worsens, they then go systemically to the heart, liver, and kidneys, creating many of the symptoms listed on the next page. (These are hearty organs where disorder can fester for years before suddenly manifesting as a heart attack or kidney malfunction, for example.)

While yeast prefer moist, dark environments such as the birth canal, they can live on the skin, and that includes the foreskin of a man's penis and on his scrotum. If a man and woman show signs of having weak immune systems (chronic fatigue, AIDS, cancer), and symptoms of candidiasis persist, they are most likely passing the candida back and forth. It will be essential, then, for both to follow the Body Ecology Diet to improve their health.

Dr. Crook lists several common symptoms in men that suggest candidiasis:

- Food, chemical, and inhalant allergies
- Persistent jock itch, athlete's foot, or other fungal infections
- Impaired sex drive
- Wife or children with candidiasis
- Recurrent digestive complaints, including constipation, bloating, or abdominal pain
- Craving for alcohol, sweets, or breads

The Body Ecology Diet works just as well for men as for women.

Children

Born as contracted, perfect little beings, children need to be nourished so they will develop strong immune systems and establish a healthy lifestyle. Breast milk gives babies their best chance at developing strong immunity. At birth a mother should be inoculating her baby with beneficial bacteria, especially bifidus bacteria from her own birth canal. However, many mothers, due to their poor diets and stressful lifestyle, lack the proper vaginal and intestinal flora to pass on a healthy inner ecosystem, leaving their infant with lowered immunity and weakened digestion. This soon sets up a vicious cycle of recurring colds; sore throats; ear infections; and digestive problems like gas, constipation, and diarrhea. With a systemic infection like candida and lowered immunity, babies are being foolishly vaccinated by parents playing the game of Russian roulette, hoping their child is not the one who succumbs to autism.

Almost all children born today enter this world with yeast overgrowth. The chronic candidiasis infection in a pregnant mother becomes acute during her pregnancy, and she will pass this infection on to the baby in her womb. Right now, a whole new generation of teens and adults in their 20s have serious, undiagnosed yeast infections. Their immune systems and endocrine glands are weak. Millions of them suffer from fatigue, depression, irritability, mood swings, allergies, acne, and digestive problems; and they have strong, uncontrollable cravings for sugars. These young adults are the future parents of our next generation.

What Can Be Done to Help?

It is vitally important that our children receive the help they need through diet, education, and emotional support in order to conquer the systemic yeast infection they are born with. Of course, they can't do this without the help of educated parents, teachers, and doctors. They must establish (perhaps for the first time) a new inner ecological world where friendly bacteria thrive. How will they do this?

First, we must stop using antibiotics so carelessly and be extremely mindful of their serious side effects.

Second, when babies are born, parents should be focused on establishing a hardy inner ecology in their digestive tracts. This starts with healthy mothers inoculating their baby with lots of friendly bacteria as they are being born and then giving them tiny amounts of probiotic liquids and supplements shortly after birth.

Pregnant women will be well nourished on the Body Ecology Diet. The Diet is rich in nutrient-dense foods; and they will be eating lots of cultured foods, and taking probiotic supplements before, during, and after the pregnancy.

Remember, inside the mother's womb, a baby has no inner ecosystem. If the baby receives those first bacteria from a mother who has an abundant supply of her own, in a few months the baby will have a mature ecological system, too. Nursing mothers of colicky babies have gotten relief from many sleepless nights just by eating raw cultured vegetables, taking large amounts of probiotics, and also giving the babies tiny spoonfuls of the juice of cultured vegetables. Probiotic supplements, such as *Bifidus infantis* (Life Start from Natren) and later, Probiotic All-Flora powder by New Chapter can be given to babies and toddlers by bottle. As we mentioned, in Russia babies are given milk kefir diluted with water at the age of four months to ensure healthy immune and hardy inner ecosystems.

Once babies' digestive tracts are flourishing, their teeth have come in, and they can handle foods other than milk, they should be introduced first to raw, pureed fruits, especially mashed berries. Bananas, figs, peaches, pears, etc., are too sweet. A wide variety of pureed raw and cooked vegetables (which are very easy to digest) will become their most important first foods, but when you feel your baby is ready for foods that are more filling, serve your little one the soaked and sprouted B.E.D. grains.

Following the food-combining rules is very important. Fruit should be eaten on an empty stomach but combine well with protein fats (milk kefir, young coconut spoon-meat and kefir cheese, and avocado). Grains and vegetables can be eaten together. Egg yolks can be given to a baby once its teeth come in, and other animal proteins can be introduced in pureed form closer to a year. Many children show an interest in animal-protein foods once their bodies are is ready for them. Meats can be combined with non-starchy vegetables, and very important, cultured veggies and young coconut kefir. (If there is a preference not to eat meats because of an objection to the killing of an animal, a lacto-ovo vegetarian family can raise the baby on eggs and milk kefir and the baby will have plenty of protein.)

Babies often prefer the sweet vegetables (carrots, squash, sweet potatoes) for their first foods. These help satisfy the sweet craving that all humans have, and encourage growth of the newly developing inner ecosystem. These sweet vegetables are slightly expanding foods. We have found that B.E.D. babies even like ocean vegetables (pureed), especially arame cooked with lots of sweet onions and carrots.

Babies love the juice or liquid found in salt-free cultured vegetables. Since breast milk is quite sweet, they will make funny faces when first introduced to these sour new foods. But you'll soon see how quickly they develop a taste for them and eat them eagerly. A child who is fed in this manner has strong "digestive fire"; is free of problems like colic and reflux; and usually has two to three pleasant-smelling, well formed, easily passed stools each day.

Children of all ages can take probiotics; see our recipe for "acidophilus milk" using probiotic powder, alcohol-free vanilla, lecithin (for creaminess), and the herb stevia as a sweetener.

Teens heal very quickly on the Body Ecology Diet. Most symptoms clear up in a few weeks, and they have rapid improvement in energy, digestion, mood, skin, and weight. Although it's difficult, but not impossible, to get teenagers to food-combine, they quickly notice an improvement in their digestion when they do so. Overweight children and teens are thrilled with the loss of weight.

Their biggest hurdle to overcome is those first four to five days without sugar. Beverages made with fresh-squeezed lemon juice, stevia, and sparkling mineral water are a good substitute for colas. Our "ginger ale" recipe is a teen favorite. Young coconut kefir can be combined with fresh lime juice and sweetened with stevia. It has an amazing ability to totally stop all cravings for sugar. Our probiotic liquids (like InnergyBiotic and Whole Grains Biotic) can be mixed with sparkling mineral water and stevia to make delicious spritzers.

Today's young adults were born into a world of fast food; for them it's a way of life. We need to develop fast food that is healthy food. Teens also need better choices at school, restaurants, movie theaters, and any other place where they gather to eat out. Teenagers have always been sensitive about their appearance, and now they're very interested in eating better and looking better. Food education is important; they are ready for it. It is time to reactivate those old home-economics labs in our high schools, create school gardens, and put much more emphasis on how foods empower us. If we don't teach our children how to take care of their bodies, the education they are receiving to train their minds will go to waste. The step-by-step principle tells us to first create a well-nourished body and brain and then they will be able to learn.

Women: Caveat Emptor

Pharmaceutical companies, aware of the enormous profit in drugs to treat vaginal yeast problems, have begun selling over-the-counter drugs that were previously available only through a gynecologist. Competing with each other for this huge market, the companies expect to reach at least 75 percent of American women.

Yeast infections, these companies would have us believe, are caused by pregnancy, antibiotics, and tight clothing. Television commercials suggest that this problem is unavoidable and "just happens." Nothing could be further from the truth. There is no mystery at all. Pregnancy never *causes* this problem, and tight clothes only make a candida sufferer more uncomfortable. It is the drug companies, the American Medical Association, and the FDA that are largely to blame. By developing stronger and stronger antibiotics without researching their long-term effects, these companies feed upon our fears, our desire to avoid suffering, and our lack of understanding about cleansings.

Even though drug companies promise you a cure, drugs will not correct candidiasis. Using them is dangerous and a waste of time and money. What you are learning in this book is a solution. You must starve the yeast until they die down to a level where they no longer can present a problem, *and* you must reestablish a balanced ecology within you. The right foods, the use of probiotics, and cultured foods (apple cider vinegar, kefir, and cultured vegetables) will do it.

Candidiasis in the colon is relatively easy to cure when it first begins. We can use colonics and enemas to flush it out; and we can eat cultured foods and probiotics to reestablish a new inner ecosystem. But once it leaves the colon and becomes systemic, it becomes a serious problem. There is no way to get into the body and scrub away yeast that has begun massing around your heart, lungs, sinuses, brain, liver, sexual organs, and nervous system. It is the job of the immune system to conquer the spreading infection. The immune system knows how to do this, but it must have the strength. That's why it's critical to restore and rebuild the immune system with nourishing foods, and eliminate any toxins that may be weakening it. In addition, women must nourish their adrenals and thyroid to balance their hormones.

❧

Chapter 20

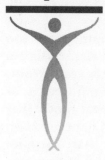

How to Strengthen Your Immunity

Since your weakened immune system allowed your candida to overpopulate in the first place, it is essential to strengthen your system in order to restore a healthy balance. There are many ways to do this; all are important to regaining your health.

• **Welcome the cleansings your body will go through.** As you begin the Body Ecology Diet, the first three weeks (and probably the first few days) will be the most difficult. As the toxins start leaving your body because you are no longer feeding the yeast, they create symptoms that mock candidiasis itself. You may feel fuzzy-headed and weak, with flu-like symptoms. IT IS VITAL TO CLEANSE YOUR COLON AND STAY WITH THE DIET DURING THIS PERIOD, and you will emerge stronger and healthier.

Our bodies were designed to cleanse *throughout* our lives— each cleansing signifies the underlying health and vitality that we cherish. Some cleansings last a day or two; some last much longer. Just remember to rely on the basic Body Ecology Diet and the techniques and products we recommend, and you will feel better when the cleansing concludes.

- **Eat appropriately for your improving condition.** As you start feeling better and better, you'll be very excited, and you'll be tempted to return to some of those "old" ways of eating—relying on sugar, poor food combining, and too many contracting foods. Or you may want to reintroduce a food, such as fruit or sweet potatoes, before you're really ready. Resist those temptations! You should be symptom free for at least three months before you try to reintroduce foods that are not on the basic Body Ecology Diet. (See Chapter 22, on introducing new foods.) Just enjoy the health that The Diet brings, experiment with new recipes, and establish this new foundation of healthy eating that will last a lifetime.

- **Control the yeast.** Be sure to avoid feeding the yeast in your system. Follow the Body Ecology Diet very strictly for three months. Clean your colon and then recolonize the friendly bacteria in your digestive tract by eating and drinking probiotic foods and supplements. Some probiotic supplements on the market are far superior to others. New Chapter offers five excellent probiotic supplements: Probiotic Anti-aging, Probiotic Colon, Probiotic Immunity, Probiotic Cleanse, and Probiotic All-Flora. Probiotic supplements are best taken with probiotic foods and with simple meals. For example, take them with your green smoothie, your Vitality SuperGeen drink, or with milk kefir or young coconut kefir.

Probiotic supplements can be taken off and on throughout your life to ensure that a variety of friendly microorganisms live inside you, but cultured foods should be eaten every day for the rest of your life. You can eat or drink them with every meal throughout the day. Friendly bacteria are also naturally present in organic fruits and vegetables, fresh raw dairy from grass-fed cows, and the fermented foods and beverages we recommend on the Body Ecology Diet.

Body Ecology has introduced several new *non-dairy* fermented beverages and a new 100% fermented protein powder to the American marketplace. These products supply hardy, first-generation strains of beneficial microflora from plants grown in nutrient-rich soils to build immunity and nourish the digestive tract.

Coco Biotic is a liquid probiotic fermented with coconut water. **Innergy Biotic** is considered by many to be our best-tasting probiotic liquid and is Donna's favorite. **Dong quai** touts the amazing hormone-balancing properties of a cherished Chinese herb known as the "female ginseng," which has also been proven to support men's fertility and prostate health. Our **Whole Grains Biotic** is made from whole grains including glutinous grains like wheat, barley, and oats. However, after the microflora break down the protein in these grains, the finished product is not only gluten free but enables the digestive tract to adapt to one day incorporating them into the diet again.

With a small amount of any of these probiotic liquids, you can create an excellent substitute for soda. Just combine a few ounces with a small amount of sparkling mineral water and sweeten with stevia to taste.

Potent Proteins is 50% fermented spirulina and 50% millet, quinoa, biodynamic brown rice, and flax seeds. Only 1/2 teaspoon twice a day (first thing in the morning and around 4 in the afternoon) will really give you an excellent energy boost. Since fermenting increases the bio-availablity of foods, Potent Proteins provides you with superior, immediatelyassimilated nutrients. See our website, **www.bodyecology.com**, for more information or to purchase these new probiotic foods.

• **Exercising** on a mini-trampoline (rebounder) is particularly stimulating to the immune system and a great way to tone your muscles. It is an ideal form of exercise for all blood types because it requires so little energy but quickly rebuilds the immune system and trains each muscle in a fraction of the time of a visit to the gym. Three minutes of intense rebounding is equivalent to ten minutes of jogging! It stimulates the T-cells, which help the body fight foreign invaders. You don't have to do a full aerobic workout on a mini-trampoline. Five minutes once or twice a day will suffice. Even a low-impact workout of lightly raising your heels pays huge dividends. Gentle bouncing, even when you feel weak, is valuable in increasing oxygen to your cells, invigorating the body mentally and physically, and reducing unfriendly bacteria.

There is a big difference in the quality of rebounders. The newest generation use elastic bungee bands instead of springs, providing a smoother, more effective session. We are constantly researching to find the best the market has to offer. Please visit our Recommended Products page at **www.bodyecology.com**

to find out which rebounder gets the Body Ecology stamp of approval.

A final reminder: do not exercise when you're in the middle of a strong cleansing. It's more important to give your body time to rest. Cleansing takes strength, so save your strength during this period, and resume your exercise program when the cleansing ends.

In conclusion, JUST DO IT. Just decide that exercise is vital to your health, and commit yourself to a new life pattern that incorporates exercise. If you can, find a buddy to exercise with—that makes it more fun and gives you a better chance of sticking with your program. If you are already exercising at least several times per week, congratulations. Keep up the good work.

- **Manage the stress in your life.** There are many ways to do this—many books, courses, and people with advice. But the first step is to acknowledge that the stress does need to be managed, to acknowledge that you do need help. If you've been trying to handle it all yourself, try looking outside yourself for the solution. You don't need to carry the world's burdens on your shoulders! Find a way to restructure your life spiritually and mentally that will aid your physical healing. One very valuable tip for managing stress is to practice the spiritual art of always being grateful for everything. This is not easy to do and really does take practice, especially when difficulties and challenges appear. If you can see these as "trainings" to be overcome that will make you a spiritually stronger person, you can truly feel gratitude for them. We can even feel grateful for the poor physical health of Americans today. It is forcing us to find solutions that will lead us to a much more elevated level of health care than we have ever had before.

- **Teas** you can drink that are especially helpful in rebuilding the immune system include mathake, echinacea, and dandelion root. But there are many others. Keep an eye out for new teas that are coming on the market all the time. Pick one you love. All of these strengthen your immunity.

Chapter 21

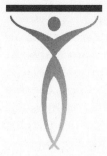

Healing at a Deeper Level: The Liver

Once your colon is clean and functioning well, the yeast have died down to a level where they no longer overwhelm your immune system, and your inner ecology is restored, many of your symptoms will be gone, and you will look and feel much better. Now it's time for the next level of healing: restoring and even upgrading the immune system to a point where it's healthier than ever. This means turning your attention to your liver.

We often ignore this important organ, but it plays a vital role in your well-being. You can never achieve true health without a healthy liver and could only live a few hours without it. In our chapter on the colon, we said that "disease begins in the colon." While this is true, it is also true that wherever disease and disorder exist, you will also find an unhealthy liver.

Know Your Liver

Weighing three to four pounds, the liver is the largest interior organ. It is a humble, hard-working gland. If we allowed it to fulfill its mission . . . to keep our bloodstream free of damaging poisons . . . we could live indefinitely. But unfortunately, it does accumulate toxins, often before we are even born.

The liver is not just a large filter, but also a biliary organ and an endocrine gland. It plays a key role in digestion, in the formation of blood, and in defending our bodies against infection. As soon as the body absorbs any substance, the liver intercepts it. The liver then accepts and neutralizes this substance, transforms it, or rejects it. In fact, if the liver did not alter the nutritive substances we eat, they would all be poisonous to us, even the nutrients from "healthy foods."

During digestion, your liver secretes bile into your small intestine, lubricating your intestinal walls. Bile regulates the level of your friendly bacteria, destroys unwanted and dangerous organisms as they invade your body, and stimulates the peristaltic activity that forces your fecal material to move through and out of your body. Bile, along with digestive fluid from the pancreas, acts upon fats, proteins, and starches, transforming them into useful substances.*

When the liver is not able to neutralize toxic substances because it is overworked, weak, and congested, *toxic bile* is secreted and courses through your small intestine, creating inflamed tissues. This is a main cause of "leaky or permeable gut."

There is no question that the liver is intimately connected to digestive functions and must be healed before your digestion, your immune system, and your overall well-being can reach an ideal level.

The liver filters and transforms protein, sugars, and vitamins into usable substances. It transforms carbohydrates into fat (if they are not used immediately) and stores it, and portions out cholesterol according to need and neutralizes its excess.

And if all this doesn't make the liver busy enough, it also maintains the fluidity of the blood by regulating its coagulation ability and thus preventing hemophilia and phlebitis. It destroys old red blood cells and helps make new ones, and helps the immune system by providing the proteins necessary to make white blood cells. It regulates body temperature as well.

---

* Body Ecology's LivAmend stimulates the flow of bile from the liver, improving peristolic activity, etc.

Signs of an Impaired Liver

Even though your liver is in distress, you won't be able to say, "Oh, I have a pain in my liver." This silent, hard-working organ never aches. Nevertheless, Chinese medicine says that the liver "cries" when it is in trouble. One outward sign of this is on the face between your eyebrows; you may have one or several deep lines and/or a swollen puffiness. A person with a weak, congested liver barely tolerates the cold in winter and may suffer chills, usually following a meal. If you have an overactive liver,[22] you may often feel feverish and find the summer months very uncomfortable.

If you have begun to clean your colon but still do not have a well-formed stool and complete evacuation of your bowels each day, you must now focus your attention on your liver.

A weak, insufficient, or overactive liver pulls energy away from the gallbladder, pancreas, and stomach—organs that play a key role in digestion. The intestines, too, are almost totally dependent upon the liver and the bile it produces.

Other symptoms of a weak, congested liver include:

- Anemia

- Hemorrhoids

- Dark, insufficient urine

- Small red flecks the size of a pinhead that come and go at different places on the body

- Skin conditions such as eczema, acne, hives, itching, or rashes; and skin that seems dirty, with dark pigmentation or spots on the face, on the backs of the hands, on the forehead, or around the nose

- Jaundice (yellow skin)

- Eye problems (loss of elasticity of lens and atrophy of cells within the eye, which leads to sensitivity to light, conjunctivitis, farsightedness, myopia, cataracts, astigmatism, moving spots, and double vision)

- Yellowing of the whites of the eye

- Mineral deficiency

- Hormonal imbalances in women due to the liver's influence over estrogen; malfunctioning of ovaries and problems with conception and menses, and difficulty at time of menopause; loss of sex drive and femininity; and developing more male qualities

- Hormonal imbalances in men producing feminine qualities, including an increase in breast size; sterility; and impotence

- Loss of weight and malnourishment

- Obesity and malnourishment

- Problems with sinuses, adenoids, and tonsils

- Alternating constipation and diarrhea

- Headaches, dizziness, and shivering

- Loss of appetite

- Eating disorders

- Diabetes

- Hepatitis

- Cirrhosis

This list goes on and on beyond the scope of this book. We merely want to impress upon you the importance of caring for this precious organ. An impaired liver cannot process toxins, so even the brain and central nervous system are affected. Symptoms may range from depression, spaciness, daydreaming, and an inability to concentrate and remember things, to more serious disorders causing mental aberrations. In its extreme, the influence the liver has upon the brain can be seen during the final stages of cirrhosis when a coma occurs just before death.

You can test the health of your liver right now. Put the fingers of your right hand completely underneath your right rib cage. You will probably notice it is hard, "congested," and quite tender. If all three joints of each of your fingers don't fit completely under your ribs, your liver needs some tender loving care.

What Hurts the Liver?

Remember that the liver is a large filter, and everything we take into our bodies must pass through it. It can accumulate lots of the drugs, vaccines, and medicines we have taken *throughout our lifetime*, and the chemicals, hormones, heavy metals, and preservatives in our food. The hormones in birth-control pills leave a dark patch in the liver, which shows up on x-rays. The fats from dairy foods (milk, cheese, and ice cream), from animal foods, and from refined oils and fried foods can also become stuck in the liver. Synthetic vitamin and mineral supplements weaken the liver, and so does improper food combining. Filling your stomach beyond the recommended 80% mark causes your liver function to slow down and become insufficient.

Lack of sleep and fatigue (from pushing yourself too much when your body needs to rest) weakens the liver. Ironically, a vicious cycle occurs as the liver weakens, because it becomes more and more difficult to sleep. You'll know you have a congested liver if you feel tired and sleepy soon after eating, yet you have plenty of energy around 1 to 2 A.M. You may also tend to worry during this time or have negative thoughts. Digestive problems may bother you late at night, and you may have to urinate more than you do during the day.

A special note to pregnant and nursing women: if you neglect proper eating habits, not only will your own liver suffer, but your baby will be born with a congested liver as well. More and more newborns have damaged livers as a result of their mothers' poor eating habits. The liver of the fetus intercepts everything its mother eats and changes it into either a useful nutrient that aids growth or one that could clog its tiny new organ.

How Can We Help the Liver Heal?

There are several actions that will help heal the liver, and the first is to *stop overworking it, by changing the way you eat*. Continue to clean your colon, then encourage your liver to cleanse with herbs and probiotics. Stimulate it—acupuncture can often be very helpful here. Exercise (walking, rebounding, yoga) is a daily must. You can also rest more, perhaps by taking afternoon naps if you feel tired. Do not, however, lie down right after eating a meal. If you overeat (beyond a stomach that is 80% full) and feel sleepy, don't give in! Keep moving . . . do the dishes . . . and expend energy until you burn off that excess food.

In Eastern medicine, the emotion of anger is connected to the liver. Holding in anger can further damage this organ, so try to express not only current anger, but release old anger that may be "stored" in the liver. As the liver cleanses, you may find yourself feeling uncontrollably angry and irritated at just about everyone and everything. Take it easy on yourself, and warn your family and friends not to take your outbursts personally.

Related Problems and Organs

Also in Chinese medicine, the liver is paired with the gallbladder, so anything that strengthens one strengthens the other. In order to heal the liver, all other organs must be strengthened as well. This includes the kidneys and bladder, which nourish the liver, and the digestive system (including the stomach and pancreas), which are controlled by the liver. (Remember, as the liver weakens, it pulls energy away from the digestive tract and pancreas, so often the stomach is not digesting well.) During a liver cleansing, the lower back around the kidneys may ache, reflecting the activity in all these organs. This is a critical time to cleanse the colon.

Chinese medicine recognizes the connection between the liver and the eyes, joints, and skin. As you cleanse, you may have eye symptoms such as tearing, soreness, and pinkeye (conjunctivitis), or see tiny moving, floating specks. Your knees may ache and pop, especially when you first wake up in the morning. You may have other aches, as if you have a bad case of the flu; the liver area may be tender to the touch; your urine and stool may change color; you may be constipated; or you may feel very tired or sleepy, especially after you eat. Once again, any of these symptoms tells you that you must clean your colon. They are frequent symptoms in the springtime when the liver naturally attempts a major cleanse.

Cleansing Equals Healing

Liver cleansing may be one of the most uncomfortable forms of healing. Sometimes you can cause it to happen step by step at a slow pace, but if the body itself organizes a major cleansing, you may feel "ill" for two or three weeks. But this is one of the most important cleansings you will ever go through.

As we mentioned, this often happens in the spring, a natural time of cleansing and healing. The bitter-tasting greens that aid in liver cleansing are available during this time of year, and the weather turns warmer, giving you the chance to bask or walk in the sun—another important way to heal. This is a good time to take herbs and herbal combinations specifically designed to cleanse the liver and colon.

Eating Right

It is vital, of course, to eat right during this time. Rest your digestive tract by eating lightly. Eat small vegetarian, alkaline meals so the body will not have to use a lot of energy for digestion, but eat as often as you feel is necessary to maintain your energy. Often people lose their appetites when they cleanse, so if this happens to you, drink plenty of lemon juice and water and sip vegetable broths made with a kombu or wakame base. This is also an excellent time for juicing, especially with sodium-rich green vegetables (kale, celery).

When you do eat, avoid fats from animal foods. Also, limit the quantity of animal foods, or, better yet, eliminate them completely since the weakened liver cannot handle ammonia, a by-product of protein digestion. Stay away from oils, ghee, and butter, because these all slow down liver function. Eat lightly steamed and pureed foods, along with chlorophyll-rich foods such as lettuce and leafy greens, and eat as much raw food as you can tolerate. Your last meal of the day should be a light one, taken early enough that the stomach is completely empty before you go to sleep. All you may want is soup, vegetable broth, or tea.

Grated radish (daikon) is especially helpful because it takes oil and fats from the body. Leeks have antiseptic properties and aid the bile in keeping the intestines clean. Asparagus and celery are good liver cleansers. Carrots help build the blood and encourage the secretion of bile. Sipping fresh lemon juice (very antiseptic) in water or apple cider vinegar in water (one tablespoon in six ounces) also helps. Rosemary and thyme are herbs noted for healing liver congestion, and you may want to cook with them or make a tea by steeping them for ten minutes in hot water. Drink this tea before each meal. Liquid chlorophyll also aids liver cleansing.

Other Tips for Liver Cleansing

The liver cannot cleanse until the colon is open and working well, so make sure your colon is in good shape before you start taking herbs that stimulate liver healing. Liver-cleansing herbs include milk thistle, dandelion root, barberry, and artichoke.

It's also very important to *avoid becoming constipated.* If necessary, have colonics or take home enemas (especially at bedtime) to keep the colon open, since the liver literally dumps its toxins into the colon.

Large amounts of lactic acid bacteria from cultured foods and probiotics (especially acidophilus, bifidus, and bulgaricus) are critical for keeping the liver clean and healthy. Young coconut kefir has an excellent ability to cleanse the liver. One half cup with each meal, upon waking, and at bedtime is the recommended amount to drink each day.

Patsy went on the Body Ecology Diet, and for a two-year period followed The Diet religiously, cleansed her colon, and took plenty of friendly bacteria. Her health improved remarkably, her yeast overgrowth disappeared, and she looked wonderful. Then she reached a plateau and became discouraged. In spite of conquering her yeast imbalance, she found that her digestion remained poor. She was still constipated and needed frequent enemas or colonics. She felt sleepy and chilled, especially after eating, and yet was full of energy at night before bedtime. Each morning she woke feeling stiff and tired. She called asking for help.

We were delighted to hear from her and even more pleased with what we were hearing. Patsy had earned a place at the next level of cleansing, and her body was telling her it was time to focus on healing her liver. All her effort and self-discipline had paid off—she was recovering her health and rebuilding her immunity. From a short interview with her we discovered she was eating too much butter and oil. She was not eating cultured vegetables and drinking apple cider vinegar in water, and she did not know about juicing.

The following instructions and menu suggestions were given to Patsy. With the same determination and persistence that had contributed to her conquering her yeast problem, she now turned to healing her liver.

Morning

Upon rising, drink the juice of 1 lemon in 6 ounces of warm water and/or 1/2 cup of young coconut kefir*.

(If your bladder is weak, you will be sensitive to acid fruits. As an alternative to the lemon juice and water, take 1 tablespoon cranberry, pomegranate, or black currant juice concentrate with 6 ounces of water and stevia to taste. You can also take a combination of freshly squeezed cranberry and Granny Smith apple juice diluted with 6 ounces of water at this time. This is a very rich drink and should be slowly sipped and "chewed" with the saliva before swallowing. One 6-ounce glass is sufficient.)

When your appetite signals you to do so, follow the above drink with another one made from a green super food formula like Body Ecology's Vitality SuperGreen.

Within 30–45 minutes, you could have an additional drink of raw green vegetable smoothie (see recipe in Chapter 13) diluted with water. Again, be sure to "chew" this smoothie slowly before swallowing.

Wait at least one hour before eating lunch.

Continue to sip lemon juice and water, if desired, until 10 minutes before eating, at which time you should take digestive enzymes.

Lunch

Eat at about 11 A.M., or when hungry.

(Suggestions given below are designed for someone who brings lunch to work and has a facility for reheating it.)

This should be your largest meal of the day. Eat mostly grains and vegetables. If you do seem to need animal foods for energy, limit them as much as possible. The menus below are only guidelines to stimulate your own creativity.

1. Soup
   Leafy green and raw vegetable salad and small amount
      of B.E.D. Dressing (or a no-oil dressing)
   Tea

2. A leftover grain dish (sprouted grains are ideal)
   Raw vegetables and/or a leafy green salad and a small
      amount of B.E.D. Dressing (or a no-oil dressing)
   Cultured vegetables
   Echinacea tea with stevia (sipped slowly after lunch)

3. Seed paté roll-ups (blend soaked and sprouted
      sunflower or pumpkin seeds in your food processor
      with vegetables, herbs such as parsley and dill, some
      lecithin granules, and Celtic sea salt; roll the paté
      up inside romaine or leaf lettuce with mustard and
      cultured vegetables)
   Warm lemon juice and wate (sipped slowly after lunch)
   Digestive enzymes (should have hydrochloric acid
      [HCl] to aid protein digestion)

4. Eggs (cook softboiled or poached so yolks are still
      soft; eat yolks only, not whites)
   Steamed veggies
   Cultured vegetables or salad with no-oil dressing
   Tea with stevia, or lemon juice and water
   Digestive enzymes same as above (if not eating raw
      cultured veggies)

5. Seasoned, baked new potatoes (topped with cultured
      veggies instead of butter or ghee)
   Arame with carrots and onions (left over from
      previous night's dinner)
   Green vegetables or leafy green salad
   Tea

Dinner

Between meals sip medicinal teas such as dandelion, echinacea, rosemary, and thyme.

Eat at least 4–5 hours before bedtime.

This meal should be one that digests quickly. Be very careful not to overeat. An all-alkaline meal is ideal, avoiding grains and animal proteins, which take much longer to digest. Eat as much raw food as possible. A soup and salad—or a starchy vegetable such as baked acorn squash, baked red skin potato, or corn on the cob—can be accompanied by raw vegetables and lightly steamed land, ocean, and cultured vegetables. Chew very well.

To aid digestion: Eat plenty of your favorite cultured vegetables, or take enzymes. Slowly sip apple cider vinegar and water during and after your meal.

Take digestive enzymes high in lipase and pancreatin at bedtime for several weeks.

Herbs and herbal blends designed to cleanse and strengthen the liver are available at your local health-food store. Take as directed on the label. Body Ecology has a product called LivAmend with wasabi that stimulates the flow of bile from the liver. It also helps with chronic constipation.

NOTE: Probiotics are not included in this program since Patsy enjoyed making a large batch of cultured vegetables each month and felt the expense of probiotics did not fit her budget at the time. If you are not making and eating cultured vegetables, be sure to include probiotics in your morning routine.* They combine with all morning suggestions, but are best if taken on an empty stomach.

*There is a very strong relationship between friendly bacteria and optimal liver function. A lack of a healthy inner ecosystem is linked to liver disorders, including diabetes and cirrhosis. We strongly recommend that you eat large amounts of probiotic-rich cultured foods to help cleanse and strengthen your liver.

An Important Affirmation

Please say the following (either silently or out loud) to affirm your good intentions for your liver:

I have now earned the right for my liver to cleanse and become completely healthy.

༺

Notes

22 A congested liver can also at times become overactive, as it works very hard to compensate for the congestion; then it becomes even more exhausted.

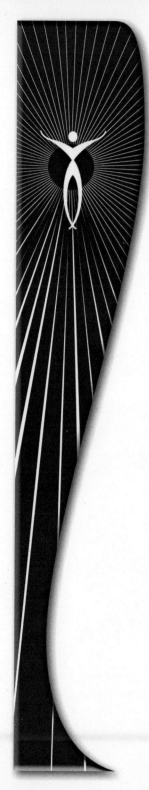

PART V

Creating a Bright, Healthy Future

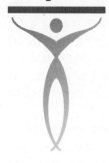

Chapter 22

How to Reintroduce Other Healthy Foods into Your Diet

Let's say you've followed the Body Ecology Diet carefully for three or four months and your symptoms of candidiasis have totally disappeared. You feel terrific, physically and emotionally, and you have a new outlook on life now that the pain and suffering of those symptoms have cleared up. You want to try some foods that are not on the strict version of The Diet.

We're not talking about going back to cake, cookies, alcohol, and other foods that would feed the yeast. Please, never go back to these. (You can satisfy that sweet craving with sweet vegetables, stevia in your teas, and Body Ecology Diet desserts made with stevia and Lakanto.)

Although you may be symptom free, a systemic yeast infection can always return quickly. Yeast is an organism that is always present in your body and under the right circumstances can easily change into a pathogenic form once again. However, you can introduce healthy foods, and by combining them properly, you can enjoy a greater variety of things to eat.

The very first rule to remember is: INTRODUCE ONLY ONE NEW FOOD AT A TIME. Try a small amount with the B.E.D. foods you know you can tolerate, and note if you have any symptoms (such as a headache, intestinal upset, or a rash) immediately or over the next day or two. If you don't have a reaction, try the food again after a few days (at least four). If you again remain symptom free, you can start rotating that food through your diet regularly.

The foods you can tolerate often depend on your blood type; so remember this valuable guideline when you add foods to your daily diet (see Chapter 25). Develop your own individual set of foods that you enjoy and can tolerate. People heal at different rates, and the successful introduction of new foods also may depend on factors such as stress, exercise, and the amount of sleep you get. We recommend that you make up your mind to ALWAYS use the food-combining rules, the 80/20 rules, and the other five principles of the Body Ecology Diet to maintain your optimal health.

What to Try First

Once your inner ecosystem is in place, you can begin to increase the *quantity* of fruit in your diet, but stay with the low-sugar fruits. If your intake has been limited to lemons, limes, and the juices of pomegranate and black currants, now try adding in some grapefruit and kiwi. These are such sour or "acidic" fruits that the yeast won't find much sugar in them. Remember to eat them alone, preferably in the morning on an empty stomach. Summer is the best time to expand into more fruits, because their cooling, hydrating effects give a welcome contrast to the hot weather. Other low-sugar, sour fruits include blueberries, bing cherries, raspberries, strawberries, and blackberries. Oranges are too sweet and are not recommended for blood types O, A, and A/B. When juiced, oranges immediately start becoming acidic. That's why we recommend you never buy commercial orange juice. Sour green apples are a good fruit to try after you know you can safely eat grapefruit, kiwi, and some berries. But for many, an apple, even if sour, may always be too sweet. Drinking a glass of your favorite probiotic *liquid* with that apple is wise. The microflora in the probiotic liquid will consume the sugars in the apple as it moves through your digestive tract.

The most important point to keep in mind is: don't overdo it on the fruits. They are delicious, and you'll naturally want to eat them, but eating too many is one mistake people often make. When and if you do eat fruit, eat only a small amount. And, once again, ideally have some type of cultured food (milk kefir, young coconut kefir or kefir cheese, or cultured veggies) *with* the fruit. Then the microflora in the cultured food consume the sugar, and you enjoy the delicious flavor. Fruit becomes a truly healthy food only when you have a strong inner ecosystem to protect you from the fruit sugar.

Acidic (Sour) Fruits

Acerola cherry	Loganberry
Apple, sour	Orange
Cranberry	Peach, sour
Currant	Pineapple
Gooseberry	Plum, sour
Grapefruit	Pomegranate
Grape, sour	Strawberry
Kumquat	Tangelo
Lemon	Tangerine
Lime	Tomato

EAT FRUITS ALONE or with protein fats like nuts, seeds, young coconut meat, or kefir made from milk.

Tomatoes are considered an acid fruit, and the best time to introduce them is in the summer, when they're in season and vine-ripened. Eat them raw with fresh green vegetables or (like other acid fruits) with protein fats (nuts, seeds, avocado, milk kefir, and yogurt). Cooked tomatoes are acid-forming and create a dangerous lectin in blood types A and B. Type O's and A/B's seem to tolerate tomatoes much better.

Adding Grains

Hopefully, you have come to really love the four B.E.D. grains and will want to keep them as the primary grains in your diet. (Type B's should avoid buckwheat.) For sheer enjoyment and variety, you will definitely want to incorporate other properly prepared grains into your diet. Also, grains are important foods for the microflora living in a healthy inner world. Remember to soak all whole grains for at least eight hours so you can digest them easily. Whole grains are healthier than grains in their flour form. Eating them with a cultured food (cultured veggies or young coconut water kefir) greatly assists digestion. By now, of course, you have experienced this to be true.

Replace wheat noodles with pastas made from quinoa, rice, spelt, and buckwheat (100% soba noodles). Rice noodles are fun to use in salads and soups. Rice is well tolerated by all blood types. Rice cakes can replace crackers or bread, but they are drying. For better digestion, top rice cakes with your favorite cultured veggies. When you are ready for rice, start with white basmati. Then gradually incorporate brown basmati (also Texmati or Jasmati). Then move to long-grain brown rice. Add short-grain brown rice last because it has the most sugar and is the most difficult to digest.

Remember, we recommend you never go back to eating wheat, but we're confident you will come to enjoy the other wonderful grains. Please see Chapter 25, on blood types, to learn about the grains that are best for you.

Beans

Beans have some protein and some starch in them, so they send mixed signals to the digestive system. Always soak beans overnight to remove the enzyme inhibitors. Then cook them with a piece of kombu (ocean veggie) and some sea salt to add minerals and make them more alkaline and easier to digest. Serve beans with non-starchy vegetables. The key to introducing them is to try the beans that are best for your blood type. Eat only a small portion at first and don't mix types of beans—just one type at a time. Beans are much easier to digest when they are soaked and then sprouted for about four days. Toss these sprouted beans into a salad or blend into a paté or hummus-like food.

Other Foods to Try

Add **beets, parsnips, sweet potatoes, and yams** once you're certain your yeast condition is well under control. These are very sweet vegetables and should be combined with non-starchy green vegetables and especially ocean vegetables. The salt in the ocean veggies makes a great balance with their sweet taste.

Avocados, milk kefir, yogurt, nuts, and seeds are all protein fats and can be eaten together *if* you digest them. You might want to make a luscious salad dressing with milk kefir, lemon juice, Celtic sea salt, and herbs. Most people seem to digest this very nourishing, vegetarian dressing quite easily.

Introduce nuts and seeds that will be the healthiest for you by referring to the chapter on blood types.

When reintroducing mushrooms to your diet, we suggest you select dried medicinal mushrooms like shiitake and maitake. Portobella mushrooms digest best when they are cooked.

A Final Reminder

Sugar—even so-called healthy sugar, like honey, molasses, and barley malt—doesn't combine well with anything. If you eat this, have it in a tea, perhaps first thing in the morning. It will digest within a half hour or so, and you can then eat other foods. If you eat sugars **with a cultured food** (cultured veggies, young coconut water kefir, young coconut kefir cheese, or kefir made from milk), you will find the sugar to be less damaging. The friendly flora help by eating some of that sugar. A little bit of natural sugar is a "prebiotic" and helps microflora grow. Perhaps the ancient healer who created the folk-remedy drink combining water, honey, and cultured apple cider vinegar understood this concept well.

☙

Chapter 23

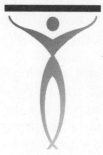

A Step-by-Step Guide to Starting the Body Ecology Diet

At this point, you may feel overwhelmed by the information in this book, and you may not know where to start. Depending on your current condition and how quickly you want to heal, you may be able to start with only one change in your diet or lifestyle—or your body and mind may be able to handle several changes. Just do as much as your intuition—some call this your "inner guide"—tells you to do. Start with one change, or a few, or many—but start.

As you begin The Diet, the three most important actions to take are to:

- Starve the yeast by using B.E.D. foods, which feed you, not them.

- Begin cleansing the colon.

- Replenish your inner ecosystem with cultured foods.

When you eliminate all forms of sugar from your diet, you stop feeding the yeast, and your body will start to discard the dead yeast toxins. You will feel hungry because the yeast are hungry—remember, up until now, they've been using you and your food to stay alive. You can eat as much of the healthy food on The Diet as you want, as long as you follow the principles of The Diet.

Another key step requires your mental and emotional commitment to The Diet and to healing yourself; this will give you the strength to adhere to it when temptation hits. It's also a good idea to tell your friends and family that you're beginning a new way of living and *ask for their support*. Then, when they see you either doing splendidly on The Diet or straying from it, they'll be able to act appropriately. Making a public declaration always helps solidify a private resolve.

Here are more guidelines that summarize the Body Ecology Diet. They all support one another, so once you declare to yourself that you're on this new path, following The Diet will be simultaneously easy, challenging, and rewarding.

- Think of land and ocean vegetables as the basis for all your eating. They are our most nutrient-rich foods, and by following the 80/20 rule, you'll always put vegetables on 80% of your plate.

- Use stevia to satisfy your cravings for sweets. Remember it will take four to five days to break the addiction to sugar and carbohydrate-rich foods.

- Only eat organic, freshly pressed raw oils. Never let toxic fats or oils into your body ever again.

- Eat a wide variety of the foods you can tolerate. This way you will be sure to get all the nutrients you need.

- Always plan meals around the expansion/contraction and acid/alkaline principles. Use the 80/20 rules to determine how much food you can eat.

- Exercise!

- Live a wholesome life: enjoy the out-of-doors, try to get sunshine on your body, and breathe deeply to relax and get more oxygen into your body.

- Welcome cleansings, knowing they are necessary for healing. Rest through them and clean your colon until they subside.

- Appreciate the opportunity to heal yourself step by step, knowing that your success will influence others to take a similar path.

- We are all creators, and as children of the Creator God, our greatest responsibility is to become happy. Create a happier emotional life by staying away from toxic people. Reduce stress by setting priorities and learning to say no. Fight negative thoughts in your life. The very energy of joy leads to healing. Take care of yourself. You deserve to be happy.

- Create more energy—you can't heal without it.

- Correct your digestion—establish your inner ecosystem with fermented foods.

- Conquer those infections (fungal, viral, bacterial).

- Cleanse—to create more energy to heal.

NOTE: Download a copy of Body Ecology's Quick Start Guide on out website at: **www.bodyecology.com.**

Chapter 24

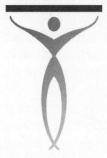

Toward a New Science of Healing

Now that you've read all *about* the Body Ecology Diet, you're ready to start *using* it. Try scanning the book quickly again, perhaps highlighting in a new color things you want to remember. We hope this copy will become dog-eared, its pages marked up and grimy from rereading and use—the mark of a worthwhile book.

Before moving on to the recipe section, where you'll find many more cooking tips, menu suggestions, and a shopping list, please consider some ideas about human beings, nature, and healing.

Healing in Ancient and Modern Times

Ancient people were intuitively aware of the inherent order, the natural perfection of the universe. Nature was not an enemy to be conquered, but a friend that supplied food and water for physical needs and beauty to satisfy spiritual and emotional needs. When people got sick, they knew how to use natural remedies to heal themselves, and they trusted the inherent perfection of nature to assist in healing.

But we moderns, as we develop our technological, material world, have moved away from trusting our intuition. We often view nature as a force to be altered and subdued, even for the praiseworthy goal of freeing people from suffering and misfortune. Our drive to create a world free of disease, poverty, and early or unnecessary death often acts at cross-purposes to the natural flow of things.

For example, we use fewer and fewer natural remedies and more and more man-made drugs. We have lost trust in the body's ability to cleanse and heal itself. Young people choosing careers in the healing and helping professions often begin with sincere intentions to return to natural ways, but get waylaid when the demands of big business and overburdened systems pull on them.

It's time to leave this track. We must once again start accepting nature's ways, trusting and nourishing our intuitive selves. We will then be in better balance with our rational, intellectual selves, resulting in exciting opportunities to create the world as we really want it.

What a New Science of Healing Would Look Like

A new approach to healing would understand that we are first and foremost, spiritual beings, not machine-like bodies that break down, wear out, or become vulnerable to attacks from strange viruses and bacteria. What appear to be suffering, pain, or adversity are really necessary lessons and challenges placed before us to help us grow. And with the guidance and protection that is always there as well, we have a greater opportunity to grow into powerful god-like beings—bright, loving, positive beings who can become powerful creators of our own bodies . . . and of our own world.

True healing recognizes a great, unseen benevolent Force that is one with Great Nature. Some call this Force God, or the Creator, or the Source of all existence. People with candidiasis, cancer, AIDS, and other serious conditions often find they improve and heal only when they nourish their spiritual selves and stay intimately connected with this Creative Power.

Connecting Emotions to Healing

A new science of healing would also recognize the power of emotions to create health or imbalances in the physical body. Until our toxic, poisonous feelings of anger, hurt, disappointment, and guilt are also "cleansed" and replaced with feelings of gratitude and joy, our physical bodies cannot become healthy. Negative emotions suppress the immune, endocrine, and digestive systems.

Cleansing them step by step in therapy takes time and could be very useful if you find yourself in the hands of a skilled therapist, but there is a faster way. If you can remember the painful experience, then find the "lesson" your soul had to learn in order to become stronger, and then really feel gratitude for that lesson; you are on your way to letting it go. Never suppress the pain. Instead feel through it until it lets go of you. If you allow yourself to really feel it deeply, it will suddenly pass. All healing follows this order. A cleansing must go to its extreme, and then it will suddenly change into its opposite[23]. After a good cry or intense release of anger, suddenly we feel light and free again. Negative emotions are benchmarks or red flags . . . signals that we are moving off target and not focusing on the rich, fulfilled life we have come here to create.

An Updated Approach to Healing

We have come to rely too much on medicines and drugs to cure whatever ails us. Even advocates of the "natural foods movement" rely too much on vitamin and mineral supplements and components of plants. There are about 60 nutrients known at this time to be essential to human nutrition. Yet even if you swallowed a mega-vitamin/mineral pill consisting of generous quantities of all these nutrients, you could not maintain your health. This is because the whole foods contain elements (spiritual essences) essential to our health that modern science has not yet identified. Our arrogance leads us to believe we can duplicate the intricate relationships among these components that nature provides.

Until researchers, doctors, and other health experts come up with better solutions, we may be forced at times to use antibiotics and other medicines. THE BODY ECOLOGY WAY IS ESSENTIAL DURING THESE TIMES. We are thrilled by the response to our system of health and healing from the medical community and from holistic health practitioners. We are grateful to all the professionals who are encouraging their patients to learn our better way.

Oriental medicine holds that you can heal yourself by eating properly. In Western medicine, the average new medical school graduate has had only about two weeks' study in nutrition. We challenge medical students to blend the supertechnologies of today and tomorrow with the natural paths of healing that have been used in the past. Young people who enter the medical profession have declared their desire to help heal; let us keep them from getting discouraged by giving them a true science of healing that is more in tune with the laws of nature.

Why Take Better Care of Our Bodies?

Why have we become addicted to foods that taste good yet make us feel full and lazy, weaken us, harm our immune systems, and shorten our life spans?

We've forgotten who we *really* are. We have forgotten the divinity of our true selves; and we have forgotten why we are really here. We were created for a purpose: to establish a bright, happy world, one highly evolved on a material level, yet governed by spiritual wisdom. It will be a world rich with music, art, and science, free from the pain of poverty, disease, and hunger.

We are moving toward this paradise, making mistakes along the way, but learning from them. Yet if we continue to eat for pleasure alone, ignoring the purpose of our creation, our minds and bodies will weaken such that we will never find the happiness that is our birthright. Once we discover our inner strength and glory, it becomes easy to turn away from negativity and dissatisfaction. It becomes easy to operate from our positive, altruistic self and take care of the body that houses our beautiful soul.

Actions You Can Take to Support Your Body Ecology and Your Planet's Ecology

- Create a demand for organic or untreated foods to be sold in your neighborhood grocery store, not just at health-food stores. Demand foods free from antibiotics and other harmful additives.

- Support the new breed of natural-foods supermarkets. They offer healthy foods, organic produce, and extensive in-store soup and salad bars and deli sections. However, encourage them to go further by visiting the deli manager and asking them to switch from refined canola and vegetable oils and cook instead in unrefined coconut oil—and to add flax; olive; pumpkin seed; evening primrose; and other organic, unrefined seed oils to all of their prepared dishes.

- Shop at groceries that are responsive to the changing demands of their public, that patronize local organic farmers, and that are constantly trying to expand their organic produce departments.

- Patronize restaurants whose menus offer the healthy, organic foods that are on the Body Ecology Diet. In Atlanta, R. Thomas & Son Deluxe Grill is becoming a well-known showplace for B.E.D. foods. Richard Thomas, former president of Kentucky Fried Chicken, is delighted with the response to the Body Ecology Diet Salad Dressings, cultured vegetables, and other dishes his menu lists. You can ask restaurants in your own area to offer B.E.D. recipes, or at least to make available a greater range of simple, healthy dishes that use more vegetables.

- Ask for healthy snacks at your local theaters, including popcorn sprinkled with mineral-rich sea salt and popped in a higher grade of coconut oil.

- Encourage schools to offer healthier lunches in their cafeterias. Participate in changing curricula so that more nutrition is taught in a more interesting manner. Students can learn how food can be fun and healthy at the same time. Help revive "home-economics labs" based on principles of the Body Ecology Diet and teach students how to cook our great-tasting recipes.

- Buy foods and products that help save the environment, rather than destroy it. Putting a serving of meat on your table requires much more of the world's valuable energy and resources than a serving of fish; grains and vegetables use even less.

- Within reason, avoid medicines that suppress your natural healing and cleansing and thus weaken the immune system. Rely on diet, exercise, and good mental attitudes to stay healthy. Emphasize prevention and wellness.

- Create or build a community of people committed to this way of life, to these points of view. This will support your goals and forward your purpose.

❧

Notes

[23] The common pimple is a perfect example of how cleansing progresses. The impurities are hidden; they are pushed to the surface and continue to swell up until they rupture and heal. Even emotional impurities (anger, sadness, etc.) follow this order of healing.

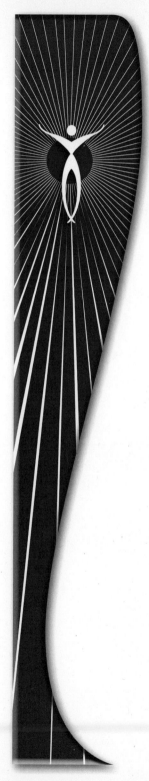

PART VI

Blood Type

Chapter 25

The B.E.D. View of the Blood Type Theory

The first edition of *The Body Ecology Diet* (1994) and all subsequent editions have included a chapter on the theory of how your blood type determines which foods are best for you. When Dr. Peter D'Adamo's book *Eat Right for Your Type* was published in 1996, we began receiving many questions about some conflicting information in the two books. Now it is time to clear up this confusion and provide additional insight from our own experience.

Body Ecology believes that the blood type theory provides valuable clues to better knowing yourself, but it is a theory still in development. It deserves much more attention and further research. We offer our own observations here as guidelines for you to investigate more once you know your own blood type. See if these ideas prove true for you; if they fit, use them.

The Body Type Theory: How It All Began

Many years ago I (Donna) met Dr. James D'Adamo, a Canadian naturopath with two successful practices, in Canada and New York. His book *One Man's Food* seemed to offer valuable clues in my own search to explain our varying needs and different rates of healing. I quickly became fascinated with his theory on how your blood type determines what foods and even what lifestyle are most compatible with you. It made sense to me that different blood types would react to certain substances in food differently. After all, blood is the fundamental source of nourishment for the body. One blood type might need more of a particular element (like certain fats or minerals) than another type would. The idea that "one diet fits all" is a bit too simplistic.

When James's son Peter D'Adamo wrote his best-selling book *Eat Right for Your Type*, I was pleased that more of the D'Adamo theory was now available to others. (Peter has since written more books on this topic.)

While the father created his theory by carefully observing his patients and noting certain patterns emerging when his patients ate different foods, the son chose to use more scientific methods. He tested the activity of lectins (proteins found in foods) and studied whether they are compatible with the individual blood types. In fact, he found that eating foods that contain the wrong lectins for your blood type can lead to weight gain, early aging, and immune disorders. Linda and I credit much of what we present in this chapter to Peter's research.

Over the years, I, too, have gathered information and observed that much of what both D'Adamos discovered seems to be quite accurate, especially regarding our need for exercise and for certain types and amounts of protein. But neither father nor son adapted their research and dietary recommendations for someone with candidiasis, acidic conditions, fungal infections, or any other serious immune disorders. Also, there is no focus on building a healthy inner ecosystem on the blood type diet, as there is on the Body Ecology Diet.

It is interesting to note that in Japan, extensive research has been conducted on *personality* and blood type, and quite a few books are available on the findings. Some companies in Japan hire and promote their employees based on blood type.

A Simplified Explanation:
How the Blood Type Theory Works

When a foreign invader of any kind enters the bloodstream, antibodies are created immediately. If the invader is a virus, bacteria, fungus, or a parasite, the antibodies basically grab hold of all the invaders, cause them to become very sticky, and "glue" or clump them together so they are easier to eliminate. As Peter D'Adamo says, it is "rather like handcuffing criminals together; they become far less dangerous than when they are allowed to move around freely. The antibodies herd the undesirables together for easy identification and disposal." While this gluing, clumping, sticky phenomenon is good, there are times when it becomes dangerous.

All foods contain proteins called lectins, which have this same sticky, glue-like quality. As Peter so well explains, when you eat a food containing protein lectins that are incompatible with your blood type, the lectins target an organ or body system (kidney, liver, brain, stomach, etc.) and erroneously glue together blood cells in that area. This leads to serious health problems.

For example, in the stomach and intestines, the incompatible "enemy" lectin becomes sticky, stays intact, and doesn't get digested. It then interacts negatively with the mucus lining of your digestive tract, creating a permeable gut and inflammation in the bowel. If the "invader" protein lectin then leaks from your gut and is absorbed into your bloodstream, it can settle someplace else in your body, clumping cells together in that region, and then they, too, are targeted for destruction.

This clumping can cause many other problems, including food allergies and hardening of the liver (cirrhosis). It can block the flow of blood through the kidneys, lead to adult-onset diabetes and other blood sugar problems, and may cause you to age prematurely and gain weight. The wrong protein lectins for your blood type will also cause white blood cells to reproduce abnormally; a high white blood cell count is a sign of disease.

Nervous tissue is especially sensitive to the effect of the wrong lectins for your blood type. Eating the wrong foods can actually make you jumpy or nervous. If you face a more serious condition affecting your nerves (ADD/ADHD, autism,

Alzheimer's, MS, or Parkinson's), eliminating the foods that are wrong for your blood type should be a part of any protocol to help you become well.

Major Points of Disagreement Between the B.E.D. and *Eat Right for Your Type*

We are deeply grateful for the research the D'Adamos have conducted that calls attention to our individual differences, but we feel the Body Ecology Diet goes even further to help you know yourself and care for your body. Here are the areas of divergence.

- **Cultured foods:** The blood type diet (BT) does not emphasize the importance of eating cultured foods, which we believe are critical to building and maintaining a healthy inner ecosystem. Cultured foods enhance the nutrient content and help the digestion of any food they're eaten with, regardless of blood type. Healing requires more protein, so when you begin the B.E.D. and start eating more protein, you want to be sure you're digesting whatever protein you're taking in. Cultured veggies ensure this.

- **Protein and Vegetarians:** BT recommends protein for Type O's and B's, but provides no protein guidelines for Type O's and B's who are also vegetarians. If you're a Type O or B, or a vegetarian of any blood type and need to take in more protein as you begin the B.E.D., eating cultured foods, even with non-animal sources of protein, will enhance the protein that you do absorb.

- **Pickles:** BT also advises some blood types to avoid pickled foods because they severely irritate the stomach lining. They do indeed. We do not recommend pickled foods for any blood type; most are made with refined salt and sugar. Pickles and cultured foods are worlds apart.

- **Food Combining:** BT menu plans show no awareness of the value in following the principle of food combining.

- **Apple Cider Vinegar:** Peter tells all blood types to avoid apple cider vinegar. We strongly disagree. This fermented food is highly medicinal and alkalizing.

- **New Foods:** BT does not include some B.E.D. foods, such as stevia and ocean vegetables.

- **Food Preparation:** BT does not include ways to handle some foods that would make them acceptable even if they're not highly recommended for your blood type. For example, almonds are on the "neutral" list for the major blood types, but when you soak them as we recommend, they are digested better and become a more valuable source of vegetarian protein. And you'll read below that while Peter D'Adamo tells Type O's and A's not to eat members of the cabbage family, B.E.D. tells you to *culture* them and enjoy to your heart's content!

- **Yeast Builders:** BT allows foods that feed yeast, such as Ezekiel and Essene bread, fruits, chocolate, molasses, barley malt, apple butter, jams, jelly, peanuts, coffee, wine, and other alcohol. On the blood type diet, all these are suggested for one blood type or another, but Body Ecology believes none of them should ever be a part of a system of health or healing.

- **Soy Milk, Cheese, Other Soy Products:** According to Peter, soy tests highly beneficial for Type A's and B's, and also tests neutral for O's. But BT does not discuss the issue of fermentation. Unfermented soy is extremely difficult to digest. It creates acidity, so the body must call upon its reserves of minerals to alkalize this acidity. This can leach minerals from your body. If you eat *unfermented* soy foods, balance them with lots of minerals in the same meal and consider them to be a protein. The second stage of the B.E.D. allows fermented soy products: miso; tempeh; natto; and low-sodium, wheat-free tamari. Body Ecology does not recommend soy products for Type B's, who usually tell us they do not digest them well.

- **Supplements:** Peter recommends various vitamins, minerals, and herbs to enhance the effectiveness of the foods for each blood type. While supplements may be useful over a short period of time, we believe that once you reestablish your inner ecosystem, you can get all the vitamins and minerals you need from food itself. Let your food be your medicine.

- **Calcium:** Peter suggests that Type O's (and to some extent Type A's) get their calcium from supplements instead of dairy products. But many people (including Peter) believe that if you avoid dairy products, you will become deficient in calcium. We strongly disagree, especially if you are focusing on creating a healthy inner ecosystem. Why? Because the wonderful microflora in the gut have the ability to change one mineral into another through a process called "biological transmutation." They can actually take silica and change it into calcium. So eating silica-rich foods such as red bell peppers, okra, or the herb horsetail can give you calcium. A clean, strong liver greatly aids the microflora in this magical process, and of course, beneficial microflora and good yeast also keep the liver clean and healthy. Other sources of calcium on the B.E.D. include dark green leafy vegetables (kale, turnip greens, collards), almonds, ocean vegetables, and young coconut water kefir.

- **Dairy, Allergies, and Food Intolerances:** Peter distinguishes a food allergy—an immune-system reaction to a specific food—from a food intolerance or sensitivity—a digestive reaction to that food. Dairy provides a good example. Many people may think of themselves as lactose intolerant, but all they really need are dairy-loving bacteria that enable them to easily digest dairy products. On the B.E.D., dairy-loving bacteria (acidophilus, bifidus, bulgaricus, lactobacillus, and yeast) will play a starring role in your inner world. They will help you digest dairy. Even so, kefir is the *only* dairy product on the B.E.D., whereas BT allows varying amounts of dairy for *all* blood types.

- **Wheat:** Gluten is the lectin found in wheat and other grains that are not allowed on the Body Ecology Diet. Peter D'Adamo notes that wheat irritates the lining of the small intestine in Type O's, but that Type A's can eat wheat in small amounts. However, we caution that eating gluten without fermented foods causes substantial inflammation in the intestines of all blood types. We recommend that you drink Grainfield's BE Wholegrain Liquid and all the other fermented foods to help restore digestion of all grains.

- **Coconut Oil:** Peter's book advises: "Always check food labels to be sure you're not consuming coconut oil. This oil is high in saturated fat and provides little nutritional benefits." It is common belief that coconut oil causes a rise in your cholesterol level. But research now shows that it is not the oil, but the *lack of omega-3 fats* from fish (like salmon and mackerel) and from flax seed oil that causes cholesterol levels to rise to an unhealthy level. For further reading on this important and misunderstood topic, see the fabulous book *Know Your Fats,* by Mary G. Enig, Ph.D., an expert in human biochemistry and lipids.

- **Other Oils:** BT does not mention oils that are on the B.E.D., such as pumpkin seed, evening primrose, and borage. BT does not distinguish between organic, unrefined oils (which we strongly advocate) and refined ones. You should never eat oils that are bleached, deodorized, or refined.

- **Fruits and Vegetables:** BT provides lists of fruits and vegetables for each blood type. You may want to refer to Peter's book to check what you can eat. However, we find that the fruits and vegetables we recommend on the B.E.D. work very well for all blood types, especially since we focus so heavily on the healthiest land and ocean vegetables. One special note: Peter writes that Type O's and AB's are the only types that can digest tomatoes. Tomatoes are not on the first phase of the B.E.D., but if you Type O's and AB's choose to add them later, eat them raw and in season.

Now we will take you on a tour through each of the major blood types, with more details on what foods you can eat and which ones to avoid for optimal health. We suggest you read through all the sections, even the ones that don't apply to your type, since you probably are living with someone of a different type. In addition, it's just handy information to have on hand; we think you will find this a fascinating way to view food and health.

Blood Type O

According to both James and Peter D'Adamo, people with type O blood have strong immune systems, a well-developed physique, and their basic nature makes them physically very active. They therefore have a better chance of conquering candidiasis quickly than do other blood types. They tend to be loners and/or leaders. They can be focused, intuitive, self-reliant, and daring.

The blood flow of Type O's is sluggish, so vigorous exercise is critical to improving health and feeling good. Type O's can exercise strenuously for an hour or so each day, and they'll feel great afterward. In fact, they become depressed and despondent if they do not exercise.

What O's Can Eat

Animal protein: Eat this daily. You can choose from a large selection of high-quality fish such as salmon, halibut, tuna, sardines, swordfish, anchovies, snapper, and trout; or free-range eggs. Beef, lamb, and buffalo are also highly beneficial. When Type O's are healthy, they tend to have sufficient stomach acid to digest these animal foods. No animal protein is good if it is not well digested. Type O's will also find that meat cooked rare and that raw, sushi-grade fish are easiest to digest. Incidentally, Peter has found that O's of African descent do better eating game and the less fatty cuts of beef instead of chicken and lamb. We agree. We have found that African Americans do not digest saturated animal fats well, but they easily digest the plant saturated fats found in coconut and palm oil.

Keep the portion of animal food on your plate to only about 20% of your meal. Remember to have your main protein meal between about 11 A.M. and 2 P.M. Eat lots of non-starchy vegetables with your protein, and absolutely eat cultured vegetables with these meals so you can digest them well.

Grains: BT tells Type O's to avoid wheat, corn, and oats. We've already discussed why everyone should avoid wheat. If you read food labels, you already know that wheat and corn appear in many processed foods, so this again supports the B.E.D. notion that fresh food made at home is always healthier for you. The grain known as flint corn is used in foods like corn chips and tortillas, and it is also popped in hot oil to make popcorn. Blue corn is usually the best tolerated, but if you've tried to reintroduce it to your diet and are not doing well, please give it up. However, we have found that the fresh yellow corn grown abundantly during the summer, really a vegetable, does not pose a problem for Type O's with or without candidiasis. Oats are not on the B.E.D., but the four B.E.D. grains (buckwheat, amaranth, quinoa, and millet) are very good for Type O's.

Fats and Oils: Peter D'Adamo notes that Type O's seem to have a higher need than other blood types for healthy fats. We find they thrive on raw butter, coconut oil, cod liver oil, flax seed oil, pumpkin seed oil, and extra-virgin olive oils. Make a great salad dressing using these oils together . . . yes, even lemon-flavored cod liver oil . . . and combining them with apple cider vinegar, Herbamare, Celtic sea salt, and herbs or seasonings (e.g., garlic powder and cayenne).

Miso: When you are ready to introduce other foods into your diet, blend unpasteurized miso (Miso Master made with Celtic sea salt) into your cultured vegetables or salad dressings for extra protein, minerals, and a delicious flavor.

Fruits: The four B.E.D. fruits—lemons, limes, cranberries, and black currants—are very good for Type O's. Later, when your inner ecosystem is well established, adding fresh figs and plums will be especially medicinal.

Type O, the Thyroid, and Cultured Vegetables

The D'Adamos note that Type O's tend to have sluggish thyroids. We find that this is true for most people these days, no matter what their blood type, because they are not nourishing their bodies properly. The thyroid needs minerals and medium-chain fats like coconut oil. That's why we recommend cooking in unrefined coconut oil or even taking some every day as a supplement. Mineral-rich foods like ocean vegetables (dulse, kelp) and dark leafy greens also help the thyroid work just fine. The B.E.D. is so effective that if you are conscientiously following it and also taking thyroid medication, **watch carefully** for signs that you no longer need the medication.

Peter also mentions that O's should not eat members of the brassica family, such as cabbage, brussels sprouts, cauliflower, and mustard greens because they suppress the thyroid. However, *this is not at all true if they are cultured*. In fact these foods are especially valuable for Type O's since fermented foods are rich in vitamin K. This vitamin assists in the blood-clotting process. Type O's lack several clotting factors in their blood, and these foods can really help. Kale, collards, romaine lettuce, broccoli, and spinach are also high in vitamin K. You can use any or all of these combined with cabbage to make your cultured vegetables. We do it all the time and come up with some great cultured veggie recipes. Cultured foods also provide vitamin B-12, an important vitamin for everyone, but especially for O's who choose to be vegetarians.

Vegetarian O's

If you are a vegetarian Type O, you must be especially mindful to eat more protein as you start healing. Try soaking nuts and seeds and then pureeing them into a paté with other raw vegetables to make them more digestible. Enjoy egg yolks, cooked softly or sautéed "over easy" in coconut oil, and eat them with dark leafy greens. (Cooked whites are not recommended because they are difficult to digest; we just throw them out.) Use our Vitality SuperGreen several times a day.

Here's another excellent source of protein: the "meat" or flesh from young coconuts, raw, or better yet, fermented with our B.E.D. Kefir Starter. You can buy young coconuts from Asian markets, health-food stores, and farmers' markets in many cities. While Peter D'Adamo does not recommend coconuts for Type O's, we say young coconuts are fine. Body Ecology Dieters seem to thrive on coconuts' fermented water and meat. (See Chapter 14.)

Avoid kidney beans and lentils at first. Cooked beans are not allowed on the initial stages of the B.E.D. When your digestion has stabilized and you do add them, treat them like a protein and combine them with non-starchy vegetables. They are easier to digest and more nutritious when they are sprouted. So soak and sprout these legumes and toss them into a salad, or make them into a paté by pureeing them in a blender along with a variety of raw vegetables. You can also soak and sprout them, then drop them into a soup made with your favorite non-starchy veggies.

Kefir for Type O's

Contrary to Peter D'Adamo's advice to avoid dairy products, we have found that Type O's do very well on kefir. With the exception of nursing babies, no one thrives on milk products that are not fermented, and kefir is the only fermented milk product we recommend. Start kefir only after the mucosal lining in your intestines has healed and your symptoms have lessened or disappeared. This ensures that the protein in the milk (casein) will not leak into your bloodstream and produce an allergic reaction. Also, since you may still lack a totally healthy inner ecosystem, introduce kefir's dairy-loving bacteria into the intestines slowly, allowing them to build up successful colonies and digest more kefir. This is a slow, mindful process. In fact, when you first start making kefir, make it from the water of young green coconuts, which is very easy to digest (see Chapter 14). Then you will be able to transition effortlessly to digesting kefir made from milk.

Kefir offers some real benefits to Type O's. Peter recommends plenty of vitamin K from foods in order to strengthen blood-clotting activity, and kefir fills that need. You can also obtain vitamin K on The Diet from leafy greens and egg yolks. Peter recommends you take calcium and B vitamin supplements. Once again, you'll find kefir to be a good source of these elements as well. Peter has had very good success treating depression, hyperactivity, and attention deficit disorder in many Type O's by using high doses of the B vitamins (especially B-12), and folic acid. We, too, have wonderful testimony that kefir is very calming and cures depression and ADD. (Kefir made with cow's milk is high in folic acid, but goat's milk kefir has none.)

Blood Type A

Type A individuals by nature tend to be very cooperative. They also tend to be clever, sensitive, passionate, and very smart, but they bottle up their anxiety in order to get along well with others. They hold their emotions in until suddenly they explode. Many A's are tense, impatient, and unable to sleep well. While they are capable of leadership, they may not choose it because it would be too stressful for their tightly wired systems.

Type A's thrive on calming exercise that soothes their nervous energy, such as yoga, tai chi, golf, walking, and gentle rebounding on a mini-trampoline. Soft pastel and neutral colors in their wardrobe and in their home and office complement the lifestyles of Type A's. Warm baths and showers also soothe; a steam bath, hot tub, or sauna can be too exhausting.

What A's Can Eat

In general, Type A's have an inadequate amount of stomach acid even from birth and do not digest animal protein or fats very well. Therefore, the D'Adamos assume, A's should avoid animal protein and eat a mainly vegetarian diet. They suggest a diet with many alkaline fruits and vegetables to prevent an increase in body acidity. However, many Type A's tell us that as they begin The Diet, they feel stronger when they eat some animal protein, especially cold-water fish, like salmon, tuna, sardines, and mackerel; and softly cooked egg yolks. If you're a Type A, we strongly suggest that you include plenty of cultured vegetables with your protein meals and use digestive enzymes. (In Chapter 12, see "A Special Note to Vegetarians.") Remember the B.E.D. 80/20 principle and keep your protein to a minimum anyway, focusing instead on vegetables from the land and sea.

Vegetarian Sources of Protein for Type A's

The human body, especially when it is healing, needs plenty of high-quality protein. But even the most valuable proteins create toxins in the gut if they are not digested well. You'll find many easily digested vegetarian protein sources on the Body Ecology Diet. Algae found in products like our Vitality SuperGreen are an excellent source of animal-free protein. Even our four B.E.D. grains are high in protein. Soaked seeds and nuts provide other good sources, but they, too, are often difficult to digest, especially when stomach acid is low. (Use enzymes with HCl and pepsin, like Body Ecology's ASSIST Dairy & Protein. Later, as your digestion becomes stronger, you'll want to introduce properly prepared beans and legumes and even soy foods. Just make sure the soy is fermented, as we discussed above.

Nuts and Seeds: Peter D'Adamo has found that peanuts are highly beneficial for Type A's. We strongly disagree and know they are not for anyone with candidiasis. They often have mold growing on them. Also, peanut butter and other nut and seed butters are often too oily and difficult to digest if you have a weak digestive tract. Pumpkin seeds, however, are excellent for Type A's; and almonds, sunflower seeds, and later walnuts are also great to work into patés. Remember to soak nuts and seeds for at least eight hours before eating them.

Nuts and seeds are extremely concentrated foods. Consume them in small quantities and balance them with vegetables, especially dark green leafy ones like kale and collards. Our favorite way to prepare nuts for ease of digestion: puree them into a paté with raw vegetables (garlic, carrots, celery, zucchini, kale, okra, red bell pepper). Then season this mixture with a touch of Celtic sea salt. You can even make a "wrap" by rolling up the paté in a tender collard or romaine lettuce leaf. Take this to work or school, and you'll be brown-bagging it with the best of them!

Fats and Oils: Peter says Type A's need very little fat to function well. We agree, but also emphasize that high-quality, raw fats are critical.

Kefir for Type A's

According to Peter, Type A's need to be especially careful with milk products. Here's why: Type A blood creates antibodies to the primary sugar in whole milk, D-galactosamine. The antibodies reject whole-milk products. We also have noticed that A's do poorly on saturated fat from dairy and animal foods. So Type A's should use low-fat or non-fat kefir and drink small amounts at a time. Fortunately, once it is fermented, most of the D-galactosamine is consumed by the microflora. Goat's milk may not work well for Type A's either because the fat is inherent in the milk and cannot be taken out—you can't make low-fat goat's milk.

Peter suggests drinking only small amounts of fermented dairy foods. We suggest Type A's try about one-half cup of kefir each morning (introduced in very small amounts only after your mucosal lining is no longer permeable). Some A's may want to drink it just a few times a week.

Kefir can also be made from soy milk, but we do not really recommend it. Many soy milks on the market contain refined oil and various sugars (Westbrae makes a non-fat, sugar-free version). Put a pinch of acidophilus powder into the soy milk when you add our B.E.D. Kefir Starter. This not only adds another valuable bacteria to the starter but it also improves the taste of your finished soy kefir. Avoid soy kefir or yogurt that is sweetened with sugar. Sugar in a bean product creates very uncomfortable gas and bloating. The microflora in kefir are "dairy-loving" beings, and I (Donna) feel that they may not really flourish in soy milk. I question if these fragile bacteria truly ferment the soybean well and hope future research will provide answers. Type A's may do better drinking small amounts of kefir made from goat's or sheep's milk or better yet, kefir from the water in young coconuts. This is where the principle of uniqueness comes in. Find what works for you.

Raw Milk: If you live in California or have access to raw milk, you will find it much easier to digest. When microbial-rich Kefir Starter is put into raw milk, the bacteria and yeast in the milk wake up and immediately set about destroying any pathogenic bacteria. Then they begin to consume the lactose (milk sugar) and start fermenting the milk, pre-digesting the protein and the fat and increasing the nutritional value of the milk that is turning into kefir. If we ever want to reclaim our birthright of ideal health for ourselves and for our children, we must stand up and demand access to raw dairy products. (Visit **www.realmilk.com.**)

Blood Type B

"Balanced" describes this blood type perfectly. Type B's are creative and sensitive like A's, yet also daring like O's. They are empathetic, easily understanding others' points of view, yet often hesitant to challenge or confront. Type B's are chameleon-like and flexible; they are good to have as friends.

While they have strong immune systems and a better chance of resisting diseases facing most Westerners today (such as cancer and heart disease), Type B's are more prone to slow-growing viral and neurological conditions, like lupus, MS, and chronic fatigue. They also have a tendency toward hypoglycemia and blood sugar problems, especially if they eat foods that do not agree with them.

Peter D'Adamo warns that Type B children can have extreme neurological reactions to vaccinations. If you intend to vaccinate your B child, be sure he or she is extremely healthy first.

What B's Can Eat

Animal Protein: Type B's must avoid pork and chicken. These foods form a dangerous lectin that attacks your bloodstream. However, if you really love poultry, choose pheasant or turkey instead. Free-range lamb can be eaten several times a week. Wild game and mutton, venison, and rabbit are also very good for B's, but often hard to find these days. Occasionally, beef can fit into the Type B diet. We do not recommend eating liver unless it comes from a free-range animal. The liver stores lots of poisons. The B.E.D. first choice of animal protein always comes from the sea. So focus on the wonderful variety of seafood available to Type B's. Salmon, tuna, halibut, cod, and sardines provide important fatty acids. White fish are excellent as well, but avoid shellfish, like crab, lobster, shrimp, and mussels.

Grains: Type B's do not have as many grain choices as the other blood types. In the first stage of the B.E.D., you should stay with just two of the grains: millet and quinoa. If you cook these two (1/2 cup of each in three cups of water) together, you'll feel like you've just created a whole new grain. The other two B.E.D. grains—buckwheat and amaranth—are not recommended for B's. Avoid corn, wheat, and rye.

Now, despite what we just wrote, note that when any grain is sprouted, it is well tolerated. For example, Peter lists sprouted wheat breads like Essene and Ezekiel in the highly beneficial category. Clearly this is another example of how the *preparation* of foods makes a difference. Just from sprouting, the food changes from harmful to highly beneficial. Nevertheless, sprouted breads are extremely sweet and are definitely not on the B.E.D. Please avoid them!

How about other popular grains, like rice, oats, and spelt? When your digestion is stronger, first you can slowly introduce rice into your diet. Then in a month or so try oats and spelt if you enjoy eating them. Remember to soak them before cooking them. They can also be sprouted and eaten raw.

Oils, Fats, and Seeds: As you are well aware by now, the B.E.D. strongly encourages the use of organic, unrefined oil. The blood type diet recommends oils that are safe for you to eat and steers you away from the ones to avoid. But it does not distinguish between oils that are bleached, deodorized, and refined, and those that are raw, freshly pressed, and still full of valuable nutrients. Poor-quality oils would obviously test poorly in anyone's body. Organic, unrefined oils act completely differently since they are easily metabolized by the liver.

The only oils Peter recommends for Type B are olive and flax for salads and ghee for cooking. We find that B's do well on all the B.E.D.-recommended oils. While Peter does not evaluate pumpkin seed *oil*, pumpkin seeds are on his avoid list. So you B's may want to avoid pumpkin seed oil, although, once again, when the oil is organic and unrefined, we find B's seem to do fine with this oil, too. Canola, corn, cottonseed, peanut, safflower, sesame, and sunflower oils all appear on the D'Adamo "avoid" list. Remember, almonds, along with sunflower and pumpkin seeds, are allowed on the initial stage of the B.E.D. Peter finds that almonds are good for Type B's, but sunflower seeds are on his avoid list.

While extra-virgin olive oil has heart-protective properties, it cannot supply us with other important fatty acids like GLA and omega-3, omega-6, and omega-9. Where will B's obtain the really important omega-3 fatty acids, especially when they must limit nuts and seeds? Choose from the fish selection mentioned above since those fish provide the nutritious omega-3 oils. Eat salmon several times a week, and include flax seed oil in your salad dressing.

Coconuts: The BT diet puts coconuts on the avoid list, but we find that B's do very well eating the meat of young coconuts. We scoop out this soft pudding-like food and puree it with water, and then add the B.E.D. starter culture. After it sits out at room temperature for 24 hours, it becomes a delicious, creamy food that can be eaten plain or flavored. Besides being an excellent source of vegetarian protein, young coconuts contain two special fatty acids: lauric and caprylic acid. These protein/fats are especially valuable for someone with an immune disorder. Once they are in the bloodstream, they protect us from viruses, fungi, and bacteria. Coconut oil is also a great source of these two fatty acids, so that's another reason we love it for cooking.

Fruits: Type B's can enjoy a wide variety of fruits on the BT diet. The four B.E.D. fruits (lemon, lime, cranberry, and black currants) can be eaten right away. Once you're into stage two of the B.E.D., begin eating acid fruits first (grapefruit, pineapple, kiwi, and strawberries).

Can Type B's Be Vegetarian?

Absolutely! In fact a B will feel best with many vegetarian meals each week. Type B's do have a fairly high requirement for protein, however, so obtain it from vegetarian sources like kefir, eggs, and algae (Vitality SuperGreen). Even though B's should avoid chicken, eggs are fine.

Type B's fare better than all the blood types when it comes to dairy foods. Nevertheless, dairy foods are concentrated, dehydrating, and should be eaten in moderation. Quality is important. Eat organic, fermented dairy foods to reduce the milk sugars—that, of course, spells kefir. On stage two of the B.E.D., you may want to add *raw milk* cheese to your salads.

Once your digestive tract is stronger, it's okay to add beans to your menu plan. Remember to treat them like an animal protein and combine them with non-starchy vegetables, ocean vegetables, and/or cultured vegetables. The beans that are best for Type B's are kidney, lima, and navy. Avoid lentils, garbanzos, pintos, adzukis, and black-eyed peas. Over the years we have received a lot of feedback from B's who tell us they do not digest soybeans or soy products well at all. Soy seems to upset their basically strong digestive system. Peter's research, on the other hand, has shown that soy foods are "neutral" for B's. If you do want to eat soy in stage two of The Diet, only eat that which is fermented.

Blood Types in Japan

It is interesting to note that blood types B and A are the two most common types in Japan, where soy and adzuki beans and buckwheat noodles (soba) are mainstays of the diet. Obviously, it's the Japanese A's who do well on such foods, whereas the Type B's have not been so fortunate. Type A's flourish on soybean foods like miso, tamari, natto, and tofu, and do quite well eating adzuki beans and the buckwheat noodles. The cultured dairy foods that are so good for Type B's have only recently become popular there. Even if you never expect to live in Japan, this bit of information can serve you well if you eat out in Japanese restaurants.

Blood Type AB

If you do not have an AB friend in your life, find one! They are immensely charming and therefore quite popular. To quote Peter D'Adamo, AB's have a "spiritual, somewhat flaky nature that embraces all aspects of life without being particularly aware of the consequences." They don't sweat the small stuff. Unfortunately for most of us, AB friends are not so easy to find. Only about 2 to 5 percent of the population are AB.

AB's react to stress in the same way that Type A's do: poorly. So they can follow the Type A guidelines for gentle, calming exercise. It is important for AB's to keep their stress levels very low or the immune system will become too weary to fight infections. As Peter says, your "immune system is the best friend to nearly every virus and disease on the planet." Keep the gates locked by keeping the stress down. Stress, according to Peter, can also lead to heart disease and cancer. Type AB's tend to be stronger and more active than A's.

What AB's Can Eat

The food needs of AB's borrow from both the A and B types individually, so they are a bit more complex. If you are an AB, study both food lists carefully, and watch to see what works for you. AB's have low stomach acid (like A's) and a tendency toward hypoglycemia, a lowering of blood sugar (like B's).

Animal protein: Animal protein is a tricky category for AB's. They are genetically programmed for it, but like Type A's, lack the stomach acid to digest it. The B.E.D. solves this problem beautifully for AB's since they can eat their protein meals with cultured vegetables. Sipping a small glass of kefir made from the water found in young coconuts is also an excellent digestive aid. AB's may also use digestive enzymes.

While AB's can eat many vegetarian meals throughout the week, they will feel best with some animal protein. Oddly enough AB's are more like B's in this area in that protein from less domesticated animals such as lamb, mutton, rabbit, and turkey is best for them. Like Type A's, AB's do not digest beef or pork well. But while A's can eat chicken, AB's are more like B's and cannot eat it. Turkey and pheasant are the only poultry that AB's can eat. Other birds like Cornish hens, duck, goose, partridge, and quail are on the AB avoid list. On the BT diet, A's are told to avoid lamb, but AB's take after B's in this case and will find lamb to be a highly beneficial protein.

AB's do well on many types of seafood, including salmon, tuna, swordfish, sardine, calamari, cod, red snapper, and trout. They have trouble with the lectins found in sole, flounder, halibut, anchovy, sea bass, crab, lobster, shrimp, and octopus. Smoked salmon should be avoided.

Eggs are an excellent food for AB's. Although eggs are thought to cause high cholesterol and Peter has found that AB's can have a susceptibility to heart conditions, the yolk of an egg is very rich in lecithin (see page 85). Eggs, like coconut oil, have been erroneously slandered by well-meaning nutritionists. Contrary to what you may have been told, egg yolks are healthier than egg whites. Egg white omelettes served in many "heart healthy" restaurants are very difficult to digest. Remember, undigested food becomes another toxin.

Grains: While millet is highly beneficial for Type AB's, you can also enjoy grain dishes made with amaranth. Our Tex-Mex Millet and Amaranth Corn Casserole could become a popular dish at your home. Avoid buckwheat, kasha, and soba noodles and the blue corn chips made from flint corn or cornmeal. Later, in stage two of The Diet, you may add rice, oats, spelt, and rye.

Nuts and Seeds: Peter advocates small amounts of nuts and seeds for Type A's, especially walnuts and almonds. They should avoid sunflower and pumpkin seeds unless they are soaked, as we recommend on the B.E.D.

Fats and Oils: Without a doubt AB's will find that both olive oil and flax seed oil make excellent salad dressings.

Peter recommends using ghee for cooking. As we mentioned previously, the blood type diet does not distinguish between refined oils and those that are fresh-pressed and raw. We find that AB's do very well with all the unrefined oils we recommend throughout this book. Coconut oil is also ideal for cooking. When you sauté foods, you may enjoy combining both ghee and coconut oil to create a delicious new flavor.

Dairy fats and saturated fats from animal foods found in whole milk, sour cream, and butter carry a caution tag on the AB blood type diet. Peter D'Adamo has found that AB's can be especially susceptible to gall bladder problems. Clearly, it is essential that they use small amounts of very high quality oils as we recommend on the B.E.D. Although pumpkin seeds are on the D'Adamo avoid list, we find that pumpkin seed oil works well for AB's; you should decide for yourself.

On the B.E.D., we find AB's do well with *small amounts* of dairy fats, especially if they are cultured. Once again, quality is the key. We take organic cream and add a starter culture to make a true sour cream (called crème fraiche in Europe). If this sour cream is whipped for about five minutes with an electric beater, it becomes cultured butter. Californians can purchase organic, raw cream and once again enjoy old-fashioned real raw butter. Because it is cultured, it is even better.

Kefir for Type AB's

Fortunately, Type AB's tend to have the same ability as Type B's to digest dairy well, especially if it is fermented. Once you are ready for kefir, you will find it to be a nourishing, very beneficial, and easy-to-digest food. However, it is best to eat dairy in moderation since, like A's, you also tend to form a lot of mucus. Low-fat or non-fat kefir will work best for you.

In Conclusion

Don't despair if you can't instantly adapt all these suggestions to your own way of eating. Keep in mind the principle of step by step. You are on a path, a journey to better health. Journeys take time. There is so much to learn and experience along the way. Hopefully you'll find this journey fun, maybe at times challenging, but always fascinating.

Never forget any of the B.E.D. principles, for they will serve you well. Especially keep in mind the principle of uniqueness, that you are the only you in the universe, and what works for others may not be right for you. Your needs will change constantly, but many different sources of information, such as the evolving theory of blood type, will always be available to you. The challenge is to know yourself and to find your own healing path.

Trust your intuition. Many people tell us that Body Ecology's system of health and healing just "feels right" to them. Focus on becoming spiritually, emotionally, and physically healthier and you will draw solutions to you as you need them. The foundation for everything is a strong inner ecosystem. With over 80 percent of the immune system centered in your intestines, physical and emotional well-being start right there. This inner world is a gift bestowed when you are born. It is an unseen world of beneficial beings that exist to serve you, keeping you happy and well. This is the world where you are "the Creator." Become a benevolent, mindful, and loving one, and you will have learned one of the most important secrets for living a long and healthy life.

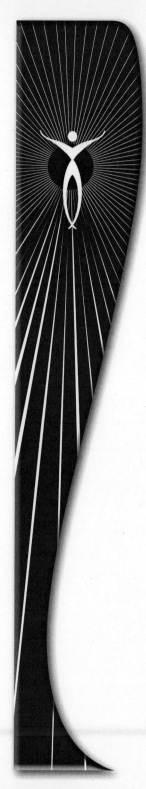

PART VII

Special Foods, Recipes & Menu Suggestions

by Donna Gates and Heidi Wohl

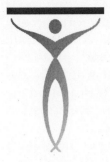

Introduction

By now you've studied the principles of the Body Ecology Diet, thought about how they will apply to your life, and are ready to try some recipes. You'll find new recipes in this section, or perhaps variations on some of your favorites. Once you master the principles, the rest falls into place.

We want you to enjoy experimenting with the new foods we introduce on The Diet, such as the grains and sea vegetables. Remember, the information may be overwhelming at first—this is normal—but soon you'll be up to speed and feeling much better.

Heidi's Story

"I grew up on the standard American diet: meat, canned and frozen food, sugar, and lots of junk food when I was a teenager. By the time I was 20, I decided I was addicted to sugar and vowed to do something about it. So I started taking lots of vitamin pills, drank 'pep up' drinks, and gave up sugar. I did start feeling better, but that was not to last.

"I studied nutrition and tried various diets. I became a vegetarian, gave up cheese and dairy, and tried a raw foods diet. Despite all this, I had lots of viral infections, sore throats, excessive mucus and nasal discharge, and chronic constipation.

"Then I went headlong into studying and practicing macrobiotics for several years. I was sure that would be the answer, but it wasn't. I developed a fungal infection around my mouth, my digestion was poor, and the chronic constipation continued. I always had a bad taste in my mouth.

"I tried acupuncture and received counseling at the highest level of macrobiotics. I was told to cut out virtually all salt, oils, and fruit, as well as many vegetables, and strictly limit my fish intake. I was desperate to be healthy, so I took all these steps. At this time I was pregnant. My skin turned yellow, I had no energy, I felt weak and tired all the time, the constipation was worse than ever, and I had indigestion after every meal. I continued to believe that brown rice, beans, and greens would save me if only I could eat enough of them.

"Then I met Donna. I began the Body Ecology Diet immediately, and when I did, my digestion improved dramatically, the embarrassing fungal infection on my mouth started to go away, and my spirits lifted. I didn't realize how much my nervous system had been affected by my candidiasis. I began to feel calmer. Things that had caused tremendous stress in the past, even such simple things as preparing a meal and getting it on the table, became pleasant. Taking a car trip to the city, which had been stressful and demanding, suddenly became routine. I began enjoying food once again.

"Now I prepare all the meals for my family based on the B.E.D. guidelines, with reasonable adjustments for individual needs. We've all benefitted from The Diet. I love to cook and create new recipes. All the recipes I've contributed to this book will add variety to your meals as well as help you restore your inner balance. They are my gift in gratitude for what The Diet has done for me. Bon appétit!"

Heidi Wohl

Tying It All Together:
How to Make The Diet Work for You

Yes, there is a lot of information to absorb, a lot of things to do to make The Diet an integral part of your life. Remember the principle of step by step. You don't need to do everything the first day. Look back through this book at least one more time before you do anything else. Set aside a time just for planning and organizing. The biggest reason people feel overwhelmed on The Diet is failure to prepare and plan. Take the enthusiasm you have from reading this book and use it to incorporate The Diet into your daily life. Here are some suggestions . . . step by step.

Step One
Take a look at what you already have.

Standing in your kitchen with paper and pencil in hand, evaluate what's there. What staple foods do you have on hand, and what do you need? Body Ecology Diet staples include: the four grains, onions, garlic, red skin potatoes, cooking oil, spices, apple cider vinegar, teas, and other items from the Shopping List in Appendix A. Get rid of foods that are not on The Diet.

Step Two

Reorganize your kitchen so it works for you.

Arrange the kitchen so the things you use most frequently are closest to your working space. For example, keep the onions, garlic, and your favorite knife near your cutting board. If some members of your family are not on The Diet, put their foods in a separate area of your cupboards or pantry. This will reduce the temptation for you to eat them, and also make it easier for everyone to find what he likes.

You might even want to make sections inside your refrigerator, with one shelf for leftovers, one for fresh foods, etc. Or organize it by meals (breakfast foods here, lunch foods there), or divide it by days or by household members.

Step Three

Start your lists.

Next, start a shopping list. Review Chapter 12 to see what foods are on The Diet, and look at the Shopping List to remind yourself what to buy. Note the foods you already enjoy and the family recipes you can easily adapt. For example, you may often serve grilled salmon steaks, steamed broccoli tossed with garlic and lemon, and a leafy green salad with grated carrots and Vidalia onion. Make a B.E.D. dressing, and you've created your first Body Ecology Diet meal.

Step Four

Plan a few delicious menus of your own, or choose some of ours.

Plan at least three days of menus. When you go shopping, you may have to revise your plan, depending on what's available and fresh. If you want to cook brussels sprouts but when you arrive at the grocery store they look pale and limp, you should be flexible enough to investigate the green beans or broccoli. Try to shop for fresh foods two or three times a week.

Some people find it easier to plan meals for a week or ten days, then rotate this same group of menus and recipes. Repeating the menu you love has certain benefits. You can perfect the seasonings and ultimately save lots of time, as you become quite efficient with repetition. For example, Monday nights might be for curried carrot soup, millet corn casserole, and a parboiled salad; Saturday morning breakfasts might be an arame and onion omelette with steamed asparagus. Put your menu plans on the refrigerator as a support and as a constant reminder so that you do stay on The Diet.

Benefits of Meal Planning

Menu planning makes adherence to the Body Ecology Diet much, much easier. If you have several days' meals, or a week's meals, planned on paper, you can shop more quickly and even prepare meals more efficiently. You know what's in your refrigerator, and you know what's needed to put a meal on the table. You can plan ahead by, for example, washing and drying lettuce for the next meal while you're waiting for the breakfast veggies to sauté. Store the lettuce in a clean plastic container, and when you're ready to make a salad for lunch, it will be nice and crispy, and you'll be one step ahead.

Another benefit of meal planning is that you're much less likely to go off The Diet on binges. You've made a plan . . . now all you have to do is follow it. You can even plan snacks so that when you suddenly find you're starving, you grab the carrot sticks you've already cut up or the blue corn chips from the cupboard. Try dipping blue corn chips into raw cultured vegetables for a great snack. Make a big pot of vegetable soup, and keep it in the refrigerator, where you can dip into it whenever you're hungry. If it's a non-starchy vegetable soup (such as the Creamy Dilled Cauliflower or the Broccoli with Fresh Fennel), you won't have to worry about whether it combines with the grain or animal-protein meal you're about to eat in an hour.

You'll also be less likely to run out to a restaurant if you have a meal planned and the food in the house, ready to be cooked. It's difficult (although not impossible) to food-combine properly in a restaurant where everyone around you is eating based on desires, not necessarily on health. Most restaurants do not offer the healing food that you can eat at home.

The Art of The Diet

Planning the Body Ecology Diet meals at first will seem strange, just like anything new. It's like standing at the bottom of a mountain and looking up at the summit. Don't despair. Soon the various elements of The Diet will become second nature to you, and you will be creating meals as part artist, part cook. At some point, you may not need to sit down and plan every single meal. You might just go to the store, buy lots of fresh vegetables to have on hand, and come home to create a variety of dishes.

Even if you cook a new recipe that doesn't taste quite right, give it another try—it may take a couple of times to get it just the way you like it. Experiment with herbs and spices; develop recipes of your own and send them to us (we will publish them in the Body Ecology Diet newsletter).

Keep the Principles in Mind

As you create your menus, remember to use the principles of expansion/contraction, acid/alkaline, food combining, and the 80/20 rules. Your goal is to create balance in your body by balancing the foods you eat. You don't want to eat too much on the extreme ends of the Expansion/Contraction Continuum; you want 80% of your food to be alkaline-forming and 20% to be acid-forming.

As you begin The Diet, you may need more protein foods to enhance the yeast die-off. You may tolerate more cooked foods than raw, but as soon as you can, try to include some raw foods, such as salad or cut-up veggies, at least once a day. You'll get to know your body very well and discover what it needs for you to feel good. If you eat something that's very contracting, such as salty meat, and you start feeling cranky or achy, you can bring your body back into balance by eating foods that are more alkaline and expanding (a salad with apple cider vinegar dressing).

If you're having a snack, ask yourself if it combines with your last meal, which is probably still digesting in your stomach.

There are several additional things to consider in meal planning. Is your body in a cleansing period? If it is, eat lightly and plan foods that are easy to digest. For example, steamed carrots are easier to digest than raw ones. Soups are easier than salads, and blended soups are easiest of all.

Take note of the season, too: if it's hot, plan lighter, cooling foods; in cold weather your body needs heavier, warming foods.

Chilled summer soups, raw salads, and fruit are cooling; hot soups and porridge are warming.

If you're constipated, avoid contracting foods, such as meats and eggs. Instead, eat the more expanding foods, such as salad and raw cultured vegetables; drink lemon juice and water. Try grains with vegetable meals, which have lots of fiber. Sprinkle flax seeds on your food, and use the ocean vegetable agar to aid elimination.

If you're a woman, consider where you are in your monthly cycle. From the time you ovulate to the end of your menstrual period, eat foods with as little salt as possible, because you want to encourage a complete cleansing, a complete shedding of the uterine lining, and salt restricts that. After your period, it's okay to increase your salt intake a bit.

Add Fun; Reduce Stress

Getting back to the art and creativity of cooking, remember to vary the color and texture of the foods you make. If you're making millet with cauliflower, brighten the plate with a lightly steamed green vegetable and maybe a few shavings of carrot or bits of red pepper. If you're serving a dark green ocean vegetable, garnish it with lemon or cucumber slices or a red radish cut like a flower. Regarding texture, serve creamy mashed potatoes with a crisp salad, or blended soup with crunchy baked blue corn chips.

Try to serve the food attractively, too. Put your grain serving in a little mold and turn it upside down on the plate, or mound it and surround it with green veggies or top it with a few sprigs of parsley. Sprinkle dill on top of a bowl of soup, or arrange lemon slices and parsley on fish.

You may be a gourmet cook who likes to spend a lot of time in the kitchen, or you may be a working mother who needs to do ten things at once. Wherever you fit, you can adapt all the things you've ever learned about cooking and food to the Body Ecology Diet. The only thing you need to change is the food itself, and after practicing with The Diet a bit, it won't seem like much of a change at all. You can use healthy cooking and eating to express your inner self, to express the newfound vitality you will feel as you use The Diet to rebuild your immunity.

Cooking to Heal

The Body Ecology Diet foods build the immune system and nourish the body and the spirit. They should be cooked with the intention to heal. A cook's vibrations are always in the food he or she cooks. Many spiritual leaders choose a spiritually elevated follower to cook for them. They know that only a well-balanced, centered person has the power to create meals with a harmonious and positive energy. Creating a meal can be an expression of love for those who will eat it. Whether you cook for yourself or for those you love, it's important to cook with the intention to heal, with calmness and appreciation for the benefits the food can bring.

Hopefully, you'll continue to learn about the energetics of foods and of the impact foods have on your body. For example, the sweet vegetables (onions, carrots, winter squash) nourish the stomach, pancreas, and digestive organs, which are often weak in people with candidiasis. You never want to cook with refined fats and oils, because your organs—already weakened by yeast and toxins—cannot process them. Excessive gas and bloating could indicate that the liver isn't handling any fats. You can alleviate this by temporarily using no-oil salad dressings until you digest the *unrefined*, essential fatty acid oils we recommend. Taking enzymes high in lipase, not overeating, not eating late at night, and using herbs that help stimulate the release of bile are excellent steps to take when focusing on healing your liver. (Body Ecology's LivAmend contains herbs and New Zealand wasabi extract that stimulate bile flow from the liver.) Blood sugar problems, including hypoglycemia and diabetes, also indicate inappropriate absorption of refined fats and protein.

As we've indicated, the amount and quality of salt you use is critical. Signs of too much salt include dark circles under the eyes; irritability; craving for sweets; and in children, whining.

What about Breakfast?

When you wake up in the morning, your body is in an acid condition after being asleep all night. Ideally, you want to use alkaline foods to bring back balance as your body recovers from the overnight detoxifying and cleansing stages. Vitality

SuperGreen is an ideal alkaline, nutrient-rich breakfast drink and is convenient if you're in a hurry.

Many people are used to a grain breakfast, but remember to balance your grain such as millet or amaranth with lots of water and some leftover or freshly chopped vegetables. This has the additional benefit of adding water to your system, which has been without it all night.

If you have a pressure cooker, cook one cup pre-soaked millet with seven cups of water. Include sea salt and any veggies, such as carrots, onions, or leftover ocean veggies from the night before; or add a strip of the ocean vegetable kombu to the pot before cooking. Cook it under pressure for about 30 minutes. This "gruel" or "porridge" is excellent for correcting constipation.

Vegetable soup is excellent for breakfast: it is convenient if already made, adds water to the body, and gives you valuable nutrients to start the day.

For a sweeter start to your day, try cooking Quinoa Flakes (Ancient Harvest) with vanilla flavoring, cinnamon, and stevia. Add flax seed oil or a teaspoon of our hand-made coconut oil after it cools a bit. You can also have puffed millet with the Body Ecology Diet "Acidophilus Milk" (see recipe), and mineral- and microflora-rich kefir from the liquid of young coconuts.

Once you can tolerate flint corn, try boiling onion and fresh corn together with white corn grits. With this or any cooked grain/veggie combination, you can cook it up the night before, pour it into a baking dish, and let it cool overnight. In the morning slice it into squares and sauté it in a little coconut oil or ghee, making a "grain fritter." Serve with a favorite steamed vegetable and tea.

Eggs are fine for breakfast, too—just remember they need to be balanced with foods that are more expansive and alkaline. That means land, ocean, and raw cultured vegetables. A cup of hot water and lemon will aid digestion.

Many people eat fish or meat for breakfast. If you combine these with lightly steamed vegetables and/or cultured vegetables, you'll have a fine meal. A glass of unsweetened cranberry or black currant juice sweetened with stevia and taken one half hour before you eat your meat or fish meal will keep you from feeling too contracted. Of course, this type of heavy breakfast would sound most appealing in the cold winter months and totally unattractive in the heat of the summer.

Include *at least* 1/4 cup of cultured vegetables with your morning meals. *Animal protein foods and grain dishes always digest better when eaten with these enzyme-rich vegetables.* No medicine can replace the benefit of the friendly bacteria they create.

Only after your body ecology is well restored can you introduce fruit. If you've been symptom free for three months, try grapefruit or kiwi. Remember to have it in the morning when your stomach is empty. You can eat grapefruit or kiwi for breakfast, then wait at least 30 minutes and eat another type of food if you wish. If you do heavy physical work during the day, a breakfast of fruit alone probably doesn't have enough sustaining power to keep you going until lunch. That fish or meat-with-vegetables breakfast we mentioned will. But if you work at a desk, you might be able to eat fruit for breakfast and as a mid-morning snack and not have other foods until lunch.

Kefir makes a perfect breakfast food. If you tolerate it well, you'll find a wonderful new way to enjoy a high-protein breakfast and help reestablish a healthy inner ecosystem. It is quick, convenient, and provides an ideal delivery system for the omega-3, omega-6, and GLA (evening primrose and borage seed) oils.

Lunch and Dinner

There are endless combinations of lunch and dinner possibilities. The following menu suggestions are only guidelines to start you on your way. As you become more adept at developing your own delicious recipes and menus, please send in your ideas and suggestions; we would love to publish them in the Body Ecology Diet newsletter or on our website. We are always amazed at how creative our readers are and how clever they are at applying the principles of the Body Ecology Diet.

FIGURE 8

The Body Ecology Diet Menu Suggestions

For the week of: _____ Name: _____

	Breakfast	Lunch	Dinner	Snack	Shopping List
Monday	Baked Eggs Arame with Onions and Carrots Green Vegetables Raw Cultured Vegetables Chamomile Tea with Stevia	Watercress Soup Summerline Curried Corn Salad Tea	Broccoli with Fresh Fennel Soup Tex-Mex Millet and Amaranth Corn Casserole Salad with B.E.D. Dressing Tea with Stevia	Tea with Stevia B.E.D. Cookies Popcorn and Carrot Sticks	
Tuesday	Stevia-Sweetened Cream of Buckwheat OR Savory Cream of Buckwheat with Sautéed Vegetables Digest-Ease Tea	Creamy Dilled Cauliflower Soup Salmon Steaks Green Beans and Garlic Raw Cultured Vegetables Tea	Baked Potatoes Topped with Carrot-Cauliflower-Tarragon Mustard Sauce and Raw Cultured Vegetables Parboiled Salad Tea with Stevia	Celery Sticks with Soaked Almonds	
Wednesday	Cranberry Juice (wait 30 minutes) Puffed Millet Cereal with B.E.D. "Acidophilus Milk"	Scrambled Eggs with Onion, Shiitake and Red Pepper Asparagus Spears Raw Cultured Vegetables Tea with Stevia	Bill and Mike's Waffles with Gingery Carrot Sauce Salad with Italian Dressing Raw Cultured Vegetables Tea	B.E.D. Vanilla Pudding	
Thursday	Soft Cooked Millet Porridge with Onions and Carrots Raw Cultured Vegetables Echinacea Plus Tea with Stevia	Baked Eggs Carrot Salad Steamed Kale and Daikon Raw Cultured Vegetables Tea	Carrot-Cauliflower with Tarragon Soup Quinoa Salad on Bed of Leaf Lettuce Raw Cultured Vegetables	Celery Sticks with Soaked Almonds	
Friday	Pureed Non-starchy Vegetable Soup Baked Chicken or Fish Warm Water with Wedge of Lemon	Potato Corn Chowder with Savory Crackers or Blue Corn Chips Salad with B.E.D. Dressing Tea	Vegetarian Kasha "Meatloaf" with Gingery Carrot Sauce Mixed Vegetable Sauté Salad with B.E.D. Dressing	Almond Mayonnaise with Crudités	
Saturday	Vegetable Omelette Steamed Broccoli Raw Cultured Vegetables Ginger Root Tea with Stevia	Salad Plate Special: Corn Salad, Cole Slaw, Raw Cultured Vegetables, New Potato Salad on Bed of Leafy Lettuce	Millet "Mashed Potatoes" with B.E.D. Gravy Broccoli Spears Sweet Carrot "Gelatin" Salad Tea	Raw Cultured Vegetables with Blue Corn Chips	
Sunday	Grain Fritters with Onion and Fresh Corn Steamed Green Vegetable Pau D'Arco Tea with Stevia	Grilled Swordfish Steak Sweet Carrot "Gelatin" Salad Brussels Sprouts Raw Cultured Vegetables Tea	Rosemary Roasted Potatoes Collard Greens Corn on the Cob Arame with Onions and Carrots Raw Cultured Vegetables	Celery Sticks with Soaked Almonds	

These menu plans are given only as examples of balanced B.E.D. meals. You'd have to be in the kitchen all day or hire a cook to prepare them all as shown. With more experience and careful planning, you can develop time-saving menus of your own.

B.E.D. SIMPLIFIED

▶ **UPON WAKING:** Sip down two 8 oz. glasses of water (take supplements).

EARLY MORNING BREAKFAST:
- **"Get Going Adrenal Tonic":** 8 oz. young coconut kefir, 1 oz. very sour juice concentrate (black currant, pomegranate, cranberry), stevia liquid to taste.
- **Energizing Green Drink:** 1 scoop Vitality SuperGreen mixed with 8 oz. water, tea, or young coconut kefir. *Option: 1 scoop ImmunoPro™ or Body Ecology's RenewPro™, stevia to taste.*

▶ **BRUNCH CHOICES:** (brunch begins when you feel hunger or desire for solid foods)
Unless you do physical labor, or wake up with an enormous appetite, it is best to eat lightly upon waking. Then wait until you have an appetite and have "brunch."
- **Grain "Brunch":** Wash grains and soak overnight to release phytic acid. Prepare a high-water-content breakfast such as a grain soup or grain porridge accompanied with vegetables. Add salt and herbs to taste. Serve with cultured veggies, or a juice glass of BE Wholegrain Liquid to assist in digestion. *When digestion of grains is poor:* Take an ASSIST enzyme (Body Ecology). Begin drinking 1 cup per day of BE Wholegrain Liquid (Grainfields). It contains grain-loving bacteria that will ensure you digest all grains again.
- **Animal-Protein "Brunch":** Animal-protein meals are best eaten between 11 A.M. and 2 P.M. Rare is easiest to digest. Combine with non-starchy raw or lightly steamed vegetables; ocean veggies are great, too. Cultured veggies are a must! Eggs are wonderful, but do not overcook. Contrary to popular belief it is the yolk that is most nutritious. Eggs are great for nourishing your thyroid. 1 whole egg + 2 yolks softly scrambled in butter with Herbamare to season; omelette with pre-cooked land and ocean veggies; eggs over easy in coconut oil (eat mostly yolks, not whites)
- **SECOND STAGE B.E.D.: Fermented Soy** (some are fine with these foods in stage one as well)
  - **Miso soup:** Made with stock using a strip of kombu and/or bonito fish flakes. A great choice in the winter months. Wakame sea vegetable and other non-starchy veggies can be used in this soup, making a very hearty meal in itself.
  - **Natto:** Buy from Oriental markets without MSG and whip it in a bowl 50 times after adding other ingredients: cultured veggies, finely chopped onion, mustard, wheat-free tamari, raw egg, etc. This is a gourmet dish for millions of Japanese.

> When digestion of animal-protein meals is poor: Use ASSIST enzymes (Body Ecology), HCl with pepsin, pancreatin. Eat and drink fermented foods *(for example: eat cultured veggies and/or sip young coconut kefir with your meal to help with digestion of all proteins)*.

- **SECOND STAGE B.E.D.: Fermented Milk Kefir**
Milk Kefir Smoothie "Brunch" *(If you digest dairy, fermented milk kefir is an ideal protein source for energy and brain power. Great for depression. Kefir means "feel good." Introduce only after mucosal lining or "inflamed gut" has been healed and dairy-loving bacteria have had time to colonize.)*
  Suggestions to add to 4 – 6 oz. of kefir:
  - 2 oz. of water and a tsp. of flaxseed fiber
  - Any organic oil including pumpkin seed, flax seed or coconut oils; ground flax fiber; raw egg yolk; beet juice powder; fermented beets; seed or nut meal; vanilla flavoring; stevia
  - Fruit juice concentrates—cranberry juice, pomegranate juice, black currant juice, pineapple juice—or fresh strawberries, blueberries, or blueberry concentrate

- **Fresh, raw WHEY:** Another great option to use as a base for smoothies, especially if you are sensitive to casein.

> When digestion of dairy is poor: Use ASSIST Dairy & Protein Enzymes (Body Ecology). Rich in whey protein, calcium, and phosphorus, this product helps build strong bones and teeth.

▶ **LUNCH CHOICES:**
Grains (soaked first) with vegetables (land or ocean, raw or cooked); soups; protein and vegetables or eggs; steamed veggies or large salad; dressings with unrefined oils.

- **Second Stage B.E.D.:**
Soaked and sprouted beans (cooked is best) with veggies and salads

▶ **DINNER CHOICES:**
Vegetarian is ideal. Best for the liver and helps with hormone balance. Ensures a better night's sleep. Examples: soaked Body Ecology grains (quinoa, buckwheat, amaranth, millet); soups made with vegetables and grains; stir-fried grain and vegetables dishes; grain salads; raw salads; steamed vegetables; cultured vegetables and young coconut kefir.

The Body Ecology Diet Soups

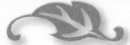

Mention the word *soup*, and most people can picture a steaming bowl of delicious, nutritious food . . .or they can remember the great aromas that drew them to their mothers' kitchens . . . or they recall how a bowl of cold soup calmed them down on a hot summer day. The Diet has soups just as good as these. They're simple to make, easy to digest, and very healing.

Traditionally, soup is served at lunch or dinner, but we recommend you eat it for breakfast, too. Because it has a high water content and is alkaline-forming, it is ideal in the morning, when your body is dehydrated. You can make your breakfast soup as light or heavy as you want, eating anything from a vegetable broth to a hearty soup with cut-up vegetables and even grains in it.

Soups are a godsend for busy people. Pull out that Crock-Pot you never use, and cook soup in it while you're out working or running errands. You can make a large amount and keep it in the refrigerator for several days so you always have a complete, healthy meal at your fingertips. When you have something like this so available, it's easier to stay on The Diet without bingeing or deviating from the guidelines.

If you don't like to cook, or feel you're not particularly good at it, soups are pretty foolproof. You can season them to your individual taste preferences, add leftovers to fill them out, and change the taste each time you make them. It's a chance to be creative and daring—it's almost impossible to make a mistake! Children—who are often picky eaters—seem to love soup.

Try what I (Heidi) call a "clean out the refrigerator" soup. Look for vegetables or leftovers that will spoil unless they're used soon, and invent a soup with them. Or make a soup using scraps of onion skins, carrot peels, celery leaves, broccoli stems, cabbage cores, and fresh herbs. The skins and peels of vegetables contain extraordinary amounts of nutrients, but use them only if they're organic, because pesticides and toxins accumulate on the skin or in the area between the root and leaves, as on carrots.

Aren't sure how to use those good-for-you sea vegetables? Put several three-inch strips of kombu in the pot when you start your soup. Remove them and chop them up when the soup is cooked.

If you have an especially weak intestinal tract, we highly recommend that you blend soups, which makes them even easier to digest. You can use a hand-held blender such as the Cuisinart Quick Prep to puree the soup right in the pot and save yourself some cleanup time.

Most of our soups taste terrific either hot or cold, so adjust them to the seasons. Our "cream" soups, such as Creamy Dilled Cauliflower, don't really use cream or any dairy ingredient; they are blended and only *taste* rich and creamy.

In vegetable soups (starchy or non-starchy), you can use a bit of butter, ghee, or preferably coconut oil. The best way to start is to warm the coconut oil, then add seasonings, then sauté the onions and other vegetables for a few minutes each in this mixture before adding your water or broth. The sautéing, especially of the onions, yields a more flavorful soup, but if you're short on time, just put everything in the pot and start it cooking.

Usually you should add salt during the final 10 to 20 minutes of cooking, or after pureeing, but if you want the vegetables to stay firm, add salt in the beginning. Add just enough to bring out flavor in the ingredients, but not enough for the soup to taste "salty."

Many traditional soup recipes can be adapted to Body Ecology Diet principles. So go to it, and have some fun!

Special Note

For especially delicious soups—and a real time saver—replace the garlic and oil in our recipes with a combined "garlic oil."

We make garlic oil from whole bulbs of organic garlic and extra-virgin olive oil. It keeps well in a glass jar in the refrigerator, and you can use it to sauté onions and shallots for soups. Doing this seems to replace the "body" found in meat stocks that chefs strive for in vegetarian soups. Often, however, these chefs resort to stocks that contain yeast or hydrolyzed vegetable protein, a naturally occurring MSG, which is also found in all unfermented soy products . . . including Bragg Liquid Aminos.

To make garlic oil, peel two entire bulbs (not cloves) of garlic and place the cloves in a blender; pulse until coarsely chopped. Slowly add two cups of olive oil while blending. Pour into a glass jar and refrigerate until needed.

If you own a Cuisinart Quick Prep or similar hand-held blender, it's even easier. Simply chop the garlic right in a wide-mouth glass jar. Then slowly add the oil while blending.

Garlic is a powerful antifungal, excellent for warding off parasites, yeast, and pathogenic bacteria. This great recipe idea isn't just for soups. Use garlic oil to replace garlic and the oil or butter in any of our Body Ecology Diet recipes.

Non-starchy Vegetable Soups
They go with everything!

Carrot-Cauliflower with Tarragon Soup

This is one of our most popular soups and is great to serve to even your most difficult-to-please guests. It combines with animal-protein and grain entrees. Make enough to have for several meals. It disappears quickly in our families.

Ingredients:
1 Tbsp. organic, unrefined coconut oil, ghee, or butter
1 head of cauliflower, chopped
Approximately 4 cups carrots, chopped
1 large onion, chopped
3 Tbsp. fresh tarragon, chopped, or 1 Tbsp. dried
    (or to taste)
Water to cover
Sea salt or Herbamare
    (just enough to bring out a delicious taste)

———

1. In a soup pot, warm oil, ghee, or butter and then add
    tarragon if using it dried.
2. Add onion, sautéing until translucent.
3. Add carrots, cauliflower, and water
    (also add tarragon if using fresh).
4. Simmer until tender (approximately 25 minutes).
5. In a blender, puree.
6. Return to soup pot, adding sea salt or Herbamare.
7. Simmer for 10 minutes and serve.

This is a very elegant soup and is excellent with animal-protein meals such as grilled salmon steak. Everyone loves it!

Creamy Dilled Cauliflower Soup

Ingredients:
1 Tbsp. organic, unrefined coconut oil, ghee, or butter
1 large onion, chopped
4–6 cloves garlic, chopped (or to taste)
1 large head (or two small heads) cauliflower, cut into
    chunks
Handful of florets separated from the head of cauliflower
6 Tbsp. fresh dill or 2 Tbsp. dried
4–6 cups water
Sea salt or Herbamare to taste

———

1. In a stockpot, warm oil, ghee, or butter and then add dill if using dried.
2. Add onion, sautéing until translucent.
3. Add garlic and sauté a few minutes, being careful not to overcook garlic.
4. Add cauliflower chunks (and dill if using fresh) and enough water to cover.
5. Simmer until tender.
6. Puree in blender and then return to stockpot.
7. Add approximately 4 cups water depending on desired thickness of soup (thicker and creamier is usually preferred).
8. Add sea salt or Herbamare to taste, and florets.
9. Simmer until florets are tender. Adjust seasonings and serve.

Variation:
1. Add 1 tsp. Desert Spice from Nile Spice Foods, Inc.
2. After blending, add sliced shiitake mushroom and cook about 10 minutes more.

Watercress Soup

Another very elegant soup, watercress is especially healing for the liver. Also excellent for dinner guests, it goes very well with animal-protein meals and is delicious with starchy vegetables and grains, too.

Ingredients:
1 large onion, chopped
1 Tbsp. organic, unrefined coconut oil, ghee, or butter
5 (or more) very large cloves garlic, chopped
1 cup celery leaves
6 cups water
Sea salt and Herbamare to taste
1 bunch watercress, washed well, large stems removed, and chopped

1. In a stockpot, sauté onion in oil, ghee, or butter over very low heat until translucent.
2. Add garlic and celery tops and sauté slowly (approximately 5 minutes more).
3. Add water, sea salt, and Herbamare, and continue simmering for 10 minutes.
4. Puree soup in blender for several minutes until very smooth.
5. Return to stockpot; adjust seasonings.
6. Drop watercress into soup.
7. Bring to boil, turn off, and cover a few minutes before serving.

Broccoli with Fresh Fennel Soup

This recipe is very popular as a breakfast soup. Fennel aids digestion. Be sure to buy a bulb of fennel that has a generous amount of the feathery tops. They look a lot like fresh dill. Use the bulb later in a vegetable soup, like the Harvest Soup on page 270.

Ingredients:
1 large head broccoli (separate florets and stems)
1 large onion, chopped
4–6 cloves garlic, chopped
1 Tbsp. organic, unrefined coconut oil, ghee, or butter
Feathery tops from 1 bulb fresh fennel
6 cups water
Ground fennel seed, 1 tsp. or more to taste
Sea salt or Herbamare to taste
Scallions and parsley, finely chopped, or sliced red bell pepper for garnish

—◦◦◦—

1. Remove tough outside layer of broccoli peel from stems, and chop (discard any woody pieces).
2. Sauté onion, garlic, and ground fennel seed in oil, ghee, or butter until onion is translucent.
3. Add broccoli stems and most of florets, reserving a handful of the smallest ones to use later. Add fennel and water.

4. Simmer until tender, about 20 minutes.

5. Puree mixture in blender (or use Cuisinart Quick Prep) for several minutes until very smooth.

6. Return to stockpot, adding sea salt or Herbamare to taste.

7. Simmer 10 more minutes; adjust seasonings before serving. Garnish with remaining broccoli florets and parsley, scallions, or chopped red bell pepper strips.

Starchy Vegetable Soups

Teresa's Authentic Peruvian Quinoa Soup

Extremely healing and easy to digest, this soup is a meal in itself. Accompany it with a raw leafy green salad or some cultured vegetables for even better balance.

Ingredients:
1–2 Tbsp. organic, unrefined coconut oil, ghee, or butter
2 large onions, chopped
2 large leeks, washed well and chopped
2 stalks celery, chopped
3 carrots, cut into 11/2-inch matchsticks
5 cloves garlic, chopped
1 large red bell pepper, chopped (optional)
1 cup peas
2 large red skin potatoes, diced
1/2 medium butternut squash, remove skin and seeds, dice same as potatoes
1/2 head small cabbage, coarsely chopped
Leaves from 1 large bunch cilantro, chopped
1 cup fresh parsley, chopped
1 tsp. cumin (optional)
1 cup quinoa
8 cups water
Sea salt or Herbamare to taste

Sauté the garlic, onions, leeks, and celery in oil, ghee, or butter for several minutes. Add other ingredients and simmer until tender. Add sea salt the last 10 minutes of cooking.

Potato/Corn Chowder

Ingredients:
1-2 Tbsp. organic, unrefined coconut oil, ghee, or butter
1 onion, diced
1 tsp. thyme
2 bay leaves
4-6 cloves garlic
4 medium red potatoes, diced
4 cups corn
6 cups water
1 Tbsp. sea salt
1 leek, washed, halved lengthwise and sliced
3 stalks celery, diced
1/4 tsp. pepper

—~~~—

1. In oil, ghee, or butter, sauté onion with thyme, bay leaves, and garlic until onion is translucent.
2. Add potatoes, 2 cups corn, water, and sea salt.
3. Simmer until potatoes are tender (approximately 20 minutes).
4. Remove bay leaves and 1/4 of the soup. Puree and return to pot.
5. Add remaining corn, leeks, celery, and pepper.
6. Adjust seasonings.
7. Simmer until veggies are just tender (10-15 minutes).

Harvest Soup

Ingredients:
1-2 Tbsp. organic, unrefined coconut oil, ghee or butter
1 large onion, chopped
3 cloves garlic, chopped
4-5 medium carrots, chopped
3 medium red potatoes, chopped
1 medium fennel bulb with stalk and leaves (optional)
Stems from 1 bunch of broccoli, chopped
Sea salt or Herbamare to taste
Ginger and/or curry flavoring to taste

—~~~—

1. In a stockpot, sauté onion in oil, ghee, or butter.
2. Add other vegetables and enough water to cover.
3. When vegetables are tender, puree ingredients and return to the stockpot.
4. Add more water to achieve desired consistency, along with sea salt or Herbamare and other seasonings.
5. Simmer 10 more minutes and serve.

Squash and Ginger Soup

Ingredients:
1–2 Tbsp. organic, unrefined coconut oil, ghee, or butter
1 acorn squash, skinned and chopped
2 medium carrots, chopped
2 medium onions, chopped
2 celery sticks, chopped
3 cloves garlic, minced
Large piece of ginger root (3–4 inches long), grated
Water to cover
Sea salt or Herbamare to taste
Minced parsley as garnish

———

1. Sauté carrots, onions, celery, and garlic in oil, ghee, or butter.
2. Add squash and ginger.
3. Cover with water.
4. Simmer for 30 minutes or pressure-cook for 12 minutes.
5. Puree and adjust water to desired creaminess.
6. Add sea salt or Herbamare, and simmer at least 10 minutes more.
7. Serve garnished with parsley.

Lima Bean Cilantro Soup

Ingredients:
1–2 Tbsp. organic, unrefined coconut oil, ghee, or butter
Two 10 oz. packages frozen lima beans
2 large onions, minced

6–8 cloves garlic, minced
4 carrots, peeled and cut in half
8 cups water
2 tsp. sea salt or to taste
Pinch red pepper flakes (optional)
1 bunch cilantro, coarsely chopped

1. Sauté onions and garlic in oil, ghee, or butter for several minutes.
2. Add water, carrots, lima beans, and sea salt.
3. Simmer until vegetables are tender.
4. Remove carrots, cool, and slice into thin rounds.
5. Purée approximately 3/4 of soup and return to pot with carrots.
6. Add red pepper flakes and additional salt as desired.
7. Add cilantro and simmer for 2 minutes. If cilantro is unavailable try parsley, spinach, watercress, or kale. Cook accordingly.

Animal-Protein Soups

Fish Chowder

Remember: animal-protein soups combine only with non-starchy vegetables, ocean vegetables, and raw salads. This is a high-calcium soup.

Ingredients: (makes 2 servings)
1 Tbsp. organic, unrefined coconut oil, ghee, or butter
1/2 cup leek or onion, minced
1 clove garlic, minced
1/2 cup carrots, thinly sliced
1/2 cup celery, thinly sliced
2 cups vegetable broth
1/4 cup parsley, chopped
1/2 bay leaf
1 whole clove
A few yellow celery tops, chopped
3/4 cup white fish (sole, seabass, etc.), cut into cubes

1/8 tsp. kelp
1/8 tsp. sea salt or to taste
2 Tbsp. parsley or chives, minced

―⁓―

1. Sauté leek or onion and garlic in oil, ghee, or butter over low heat.
2. Add carrots and celery and continue to sauté for several minutes.
3. Add broth, cover, and simmer until vegetables are partially tender, about 5 minutes.
4. Add parsley, bay leaf, clove, celery tops, and fish.
5. Simmer 3 minutes more.
6. Add kelp and sea salt and remove bay leaf.
7. Serve with snipped parsley or chives.

Creamy Salmon Soup with Greens

Ingredients:
1–2 Tbsp. organic, unrefined coconut oil, ghee, or butter
1 large onion, cubed
3 carrots, chopped
1 large daikon, chopped
1 bunch kale, chopped
2 heaping tsp. dried dill
Two 7 oz. cans salmon (including bones)
3 Tbsp. lemon juice (or to taste)
Sea salt to taste

―⁓―

1. In a large saucepan, sauté onion in oil, ghee, or butter.
2. Add daikon and carrots and continue to sauté for several minutes.
3. Add dill and a small amount of water.
4. Place lid on saucepan and simmer on low heat for 15 minutes.
5. Add kale and cook until kale is tender.
6. Place in a blender, add salmon, and blend. Add spring water as necessary to make blending go smoothly.
7. Return to saucepan.

8. Add sea salt.
9. Cook 10 more minutes.
10. Squeeze in lemon juice before serving.

Asparagus Soup

This soup is delicious hot or cold. Because of the chicken broth, it only combines with non-starchy vegetables.

Ingredients:
1–2 Tbsp. organic, unrefined coconut oil, ghee, or butter
3–4 large yellow onions, chopped
5 cans chicken broth
3 1/2 lbs. fresh asparagus, with tops cut off and set aside,
    stalks cut into 1″ pieces (cut and discard tough ends)
Sea salt to taste
Pepper to taste

1. Sauté onions in oil, ghee, or butter until soft and
    golden.
2. Heat broth, and add cooked onions and asparagus stalk
    pieces.
3. Cook on low heat until asparagus is soft.
4. While cooking, add sea salt and pepper.
5. Puree, then return to heat and add asparagus tops.
6. Cook for 10 more minutes
    (take off heat before tops become too soft).
7. For a cool soup, refrigerate.

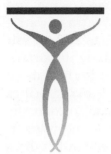

The Body Ecology Diet
Grain-like Seeds

A whole new world of grain dishes and recipes can open up for you as you explore the four grain-like seeds on The Diet: millet, quinoa (keen-wah), buckwheat, and amaranth. You may be used to eating a lot of wheat and rice, breads and cereals, but if you try our recipes with an open mind, your cravings for these "common" breads and grains will diminish.

Try to eat a meal with these grain-like seeds (with vegetables, of course!) at least once a day. When soaked and then cooked with herbs, vegetables, and seasonings, they are more flavorful and even more healing.

Soaking the grains in water for 8 to 24 hours before cooking them is a must. This makes them easier to digest. Be sure to wash them well; quinoa has a bitter outer coating, and millet tends to carry a lot of "dirt" and scum. Buy a strainer with very fine mesh (particularly for amaranth and quinoa) and rinse the grains under running water for a couple minutes before starting to cook them. You may store grains in the refrigerator to keep any insects at bay.

The basic water-to-grain ratio is 2-1 for quinoa and buckwheat, although it can vary according to taste, recipe, and method of cooking (e.g., pressure cooker). A 3-1 ratio of water-to-grain is better for amaranth and millet. You can add sea salt to the pot as you start cooking; this is particularly important for buckwheat, which is acid-forming and needs the salt to make it more alkaline. Roasting millet before cooking brings out a nutty sort of taste that is particularly good. To roast the millet, just pour it into a dry pan after you soak and wash it, turn the heat on very low, and stir slowly until the millet dries and you smell a nutty scent. The millet won't brown.

In addition to the recipes in this section, here are some suggestions for simple ways to use the Body Ecology Diet grain-like seeds:

Make cream of buckwheat or quinoa flakes with stevia, cinnamon, vanilla, and ghee—or throw in small squares of nori as it's cooking for a more savory flavor. Linda cooks amaranth with dulse, then adds ghee and a pinch of pepper. Heidi serves quinoa or amaranth with carrots, peas, and onions. All the grains are very compatible with red potatoes; and you can combine them with onions, peas, parsley, and dill. Buckwheat also goes well with corn, cabbage, onions, and many of the organic herbal seasoning blends.

For summer lunches, you can toss pre-cooked millet or quinoa into a fresh green salad or into a cooked vegetable dish served at room temperature. You can make any number of sauces, such as Curried Cauliflower or Gingery Carrot Sauce, and spoon them over the grain-like seeds. Enjoy!

Basic Amaranth Recipe—Pressure Cooked

Ingredients: (makes 2 cups)
1 cup amaranth
2 cups water
1/4 tsp. sea salt or to taste
1 Tbsp. organic, unrefined coconut oil, ghee, or butter
    (optional)

1. Combine the amaranth, water, and salt in pressure cooker.
2. Adjust heat to maintain high pressure and cook for 6 minutes.
3. Reduce pressure with a quick-release method.
4. Remove the lid, tilting it away from you to allow any excess steam to escape.
5. Stir well, adding oil, ghee, or butter if desired. If the mixture is too thin, boil gently while stirring constantly until thickened, about 30 seconds.

Heidi's Onion Pie

Crust:
2 cups amaranth flour
1 tsp. sea salt
5 Tbsp. butter or 4 Tbsp. organic, unrefined coconut oil
Approximately 1/2 cup water

1. In a bowl or food processor, place flour, sea salt, and butter or oil.
2. Cut or pulse butter into dough until crumbly, gradually adding water until dough begins to form a ball.
3. Remove from bowl or processor and form into flat ball.
4. Place on wax paper, sprinkle flour around the ball, and roll the ball out using wax paper both under and on top of the dough to facilitate rolling.
5. Transfer the crust to a round pizza pan.
6. Crimp edges.

Sauce:
4–6 large onions, thinly sliced in 1/2 rounds
4 cloves garlic, minced
1 Tbsp. Italian blend or oregano, parsley, rosemary, basil, and celery seed
1/2 tsp. basil
1 Tbsp. organic, unrefined coconut oil, butter, or ghee
1 cup water
1 1/2–2 tsp. sea salt
1/2 cup amaranth
Pinch of red pepper flakes

1/2 red bell pepper, minced

2–3 green onions, thinly sliced in rounds

1 Tbsp. fresh herbs such as basil or cilantro, minced (optional)

—◦◦◦—

1. Sauté onion, garlic, herbs, and pepper flakes in oil, butter, or ghee.
2. Reduce heat, cover, and cook until onions are tender, approximately 15 minutes.
3. Add water, sea salt, and amaranth.
4. Bring to a boil, reduce heat, and simmer, covered, for approximately 20 minutes.
5. Remove lid and boil off excess liquid.
6. Add red bell pepper, green onions, and optional fresh herb for the last 2–3 minutes of cooking.

General Directions: (makes 4 servings)
1. Preheat oven to 400 degrees.
2. Bake crust for 10 minutes.
3. Add sauce.
4. Sprinkle with Herbamare, garlic powder, and/or pepper flakes if desired.
5. Bake for approximately 20 minutes.

Basic Quinoa Recipe

Ingredients:

1 cup quinoa

2 cups water

1 pinch sea salt

—◦◦◦—

1. Rinse quinoa several minutes in a strainer.
2. Place water and salt in a saucepan and bring to a rapid boil.
3. Add quinoa, reduce heat, cover, and simmer until all the water is absorbed and the grains become translucent and pop open (15–25 minutes).

Variation: For a rich, nutty flavor, toast quinoa (with or without organic, unrefined oil) in a skillet, stirring constantly, before adding to the water.

Curried Quinoa

Ingredients:
1–2 Tbsp. organic, unrefined coconut oil or ghee
1 Tbsp. curry powder
1 tsp. sea salt or Herbamare
2 cups cooked quinoa
2 medium onions, diced
2 cups cooked vegetables (peas, corn, potatoes, red bell
    pepper, cabbage, yellow squash, etc.)

1. Melt ghee or heat oil in wok or skillet.
2. Add curry powder and sea salt, or Herbamare.
3. Sauté onions for several minutes until translucent.
4. Add other cooked vegetables. Sauté several minutes.
5. Add quinoa and adjust seasonings.

Heavenly Quinoa Hash

This protein-rich meal is a perfect way to use leftovers. From *Delicious* magazine.

Ingredients: (makes 6 servings)
1 cup quinoa
2 cups water
1/4 tsp. sea salt
1 large onion, sliced
4–6 garlic cloves, minced
1 red pepper, diced
1/2 tsp. ginger, minced
2 red skin potatoes, cooked and diced
1/4 cup minced parsley
2 Tbsp. organic, unrefined coconut oil, ghee, or butter
Herbamare and/or sea salt to taste

1. Rinse quinoa several minutes in a strainer.
2. Place water and salt in a saucepan and bring to a rapid boil.
3. Add quinoa, reduce heat, cover, and simmer until all the water is absorbed and the grains become translucent and pop open (15–25 minutes).
4. In a separate pan, sauté onion in oil, ghee, or butter until translucent.
5. Add garlic and red pepper and sauté until tender.
6. Add potatoes, ginger, and parsley and sauté for a few minutes more.
7. Fold in cooked quinoa, and sauté until heated.
8. Taste, and adjust seasonings before serving.

Quinoa (or Buckwheat) Stuffed Peppers

Ingredients: (makes 6 servings)
2 cups cooked quinoa, other B.E.D. grains, or combination
1–2 Tbsp. organic, unrefined coconut oil, ghee, or butter
1 medium onion, chopped fine
1 tsp. sea salt or to taste
3/4 tsp. pepper
2 Tbsp. dried sweet basil
2 Tbsp. paprika
4–6 cloves garlic, chopped fine
2 stalks celery, chopped fine
1 lb. greens such as kale, parboiled 5 minutes, chopped
6 red peppers, seeded and parboiled 5 minutes

1. Sauté onion in oil, ghee, or butter with seasonings until translucent.
2. Add garlic, celery, and greens; cook until tender.
3. Blend with cooked grains.
4. Taste mixture and adjust seasonings.
5. Stuff red peppers with grain mixture.
6. Bake at 350 degrees in oiled casserole dish for 45 minutes.

Basic Buckwheat Recipe

Ingredients:
1 cup buckwheat
2 cups water
1 tsp. sea salt or to taste

—⚬⚬—

1. Soak and rinse buckwheat in strainer.
2. Place water and salt in a saucepan and bring to a rapid boil.
3. Add buckwheat, reduce heat, cover, and simmer until all the water is absorbed (approximately 15 minutes).

Variation: For a rich, nutty flavor, toast buckwheat (with or without organic, unrefined coconut oil, ghee, or butter) in a skillet, stirring constantly, before adding to the water.

Buckwheat Croquettes

Ingredients:
2–3 Tbsp. organic, unrefined coconut oil, ghee, or butter
1 large onion, minced
2 stalks celery, finely minced
2 cloves garlic, finely minced
1/2 cup parsley, finely minced
1 carrot, finely grated
2 cups cracked, roasted buckwheat
3 cups vegetable broth or water
1 tsp. Herbamare
1/2 tsp. sea salt
1 Tbsp. curry seasoning or your favorite herbal blend
   (Spice Hunter)
1/2 cup arrowroot powder
1 cup millet, quinoa, or amaranth flour

—⚬⚬—

1. Sauté onion in 1 Tbsp. of oil, ghee, or butter until slightly browned.
2. Add celery, garlic, parsley, carrot, and broth or water.
3. Cover and cook for 5 minutes.

4. Add buckwheat, Herbamare, sea salt, curry seasoning, and arrowroot.
5. Cover and cook on low for 10 minutes.
6. Turn off heat and allow to steam, covered, for 10 more minutes.
7. Add flour, mix well, and set aside to cool.
8. When cool, form into patties.
9. Sauté burgers in just enough oil, ghee, or butter to prevent sticking to pan.
10. Drain on paper towels and serve.

This is a nice meal served with garlic green beans and a grated carrot salad.

Buckwheat with Corn and Cabbage

Ingredients:
1–2 Tbsp. organic, unrefined coconut oil, ghee, or butter
2 cups corn kernels
3 cups chopped cabbage (preferably savoy)
1 large onion, chopped
1/2 red pepper, minced
4 cups vegetable stock or water
1 1/4 tsp. sea salt
1/4 tsp. pepper
1 Tbsp. fajita seasoning or other favorite herbal blend (Spice Hunter)
2 cups roasted buckwheat
1/4–1/2 cup parsley, minced

—⁓—

1. Sauté vegetables except parsley in oil, ghee, or butter for about 5 minutes.
2. Add stock or water, salt, pepper, and fajita seasoning.
3. Bring to boil.
4. Add buckwheat.
5. Simmer for 20 minutes.
6. Turn off heat, fold in parsley, and allow to sit, covered, for 10 minutes.

Vegetarian Kasha "Meatloaf"

This recipe is good with Squash and Ginger Soup and green vegetables.

Ingredients:

1 cup buckwheat, cooked in 3 cups water with 3/4 tsp. sea
    salt for 45 minutes
1-2 Tbsp. organic, unrefined coconut oil, ghee, or butter
1 medium onion, chopped fine
4 garlic cloves, chopped fine
4 stalks of celery, chopped
1 red pepper, seeds removed, and diced (optional)
1 Tbsp. (or to taste) chili powder blend (Spice Hunter)
Sea salt and black pepper to taste
2 ears fresh corn, cut off the cob
2 cups fresh spinach or cabbage or kale, chopped
1 can water chestnuts, drained and chopped (optional)
1 bunch scallions, chopped fine

———

1. Warm oil, ghee, or butter in a large skillet.
2. Sauté onion, garlic, celery, and red pepper until soft.
3. Add chili powder blend, sea salt, and black pepper.
4. Add corn, greens, and water chestnuts; sauté until soft.
5. Add cooked buckwheat and sauté all together well.
6. Taste, and adjust seasonings.
7. Fold in scallions.
8. Pour mixture in oiled loaf or casserole pan.
9. Bake at 400 degrees for 45–60 minutes.
10. Serve with a sauce such as Gingery Carrot Sauce or the
    Body Ecology Diet Gravy.

Variations:

1. Instead of pouring the mixture into a pan: scoop out the seeds and membranes of 4 red pepper shells or carve out the center of 4 onions. Then fold the mixture into the pepper shells or onion bowls and bake the stuffed peppers/onions at 350 degrees for 30 minutes.

2. Instead of pouring the mixture into a pan: fold the mixture into steamed cabbage leaves, wrap the leaves in a roll, and bake at 350 degrees for 30 minutes.

Basic Millet Recipe

Ingredients:
1 cup millet
3 cups water
1 tsp. sea salt or to taste

———

1. Wash millet well and drain.
2. Boil water and sea salt. (To get fluffy millet, boil water and salt before adding millet. If you start grains in cold water, they become creamier and sticky.)
3. Add millet, cover, reduce heat, and simmer for 25 to 30 minutes.
4. Let stand covered for 5 to 10 minutes to increase fluffiness if desired.

Variation: For an even more delicious flavor, roast millet in a heavy skillet until millet has a nutty smell.

Millet "Mashed Potatoes"

Ingredients:
1 Tbsp. organic, unrefined coconut oil, ghee, or butter
1 small onion, chopped
1 cup millet (washed)
1/2 head cauliflower, chopped
2 3/4 cup water
1/4 tsp. salt

———

1. Sauté onion in oil, ghee, or butter in pressure cooker.
2. Add millet and lightly sauté.
3. Add cauliflower; sauté.
4. Add water and salt.
5. Bring to pressure, reduce heat, and cook 25 minutes.

Variation: Add 1 medium chopped carrot when sautéing cauliflower.

Millet and Sweet Vegetables

With the sweet vegetables (onions, carrots, butternut squash), this dish strengthens the spleen/pancreas and stomach. For the first two to three months on The Diet, you may find that this dish prepared with the butternut squash is too sweet and feeds the candida. If so, leave the butternut squash out of the recipe. The onions and carrots will not cause any problems. Better yet, if you eat cultured veggies with this meal the microflora will eat up the sugar in the squash.

Ingredients:
2 cups millet, rinsed and dry roasted in skillet
2 medium onions, finely chopped
3 carrots, diced
1 small butternut squash, with skin cut off, cubed
1 tsp. sea salt
5 1/2 cups water
1 Tbsp. organic, unrefined coconut oil, ghee, or butter
Several pinches of herbs such as thyme, rosemary, sage, and celery seed (optional)

—∾—

1. Into a pressure cooker, place millet, and vegetables. (This dish can also be prepared in a saucepan. Increase the amount of water to 6 cups and follow the same directions.)
2. Dissolve sea salt into water and gently pour water around sides of millet and vegetables.
3. Close cover and bring up to pressure, and cook on low flame for 30 minutes.
4. Reduce pressure and open lid.
5. Fold in oil, ghee, or butter and herbs.
6. Stir well and serve.

Variations:
1. To create a creamier consistency, puree the millet/vegetable mixture with oil, ghee, or butter in a blender.
2. Add 3-inch strips of kombu ocean vegetable in the pressure cooker with the millet and vegetables. The dish will not be as sweet, but it will have extra minerals.

Tex-Mex Millet and Amaranth Corn Casserole

Ingredients:

1 Tbsp. organic, unrefined coconut oil, ghee, or butter
1 1/2 cups millet, washed and drained
1/2 cup amaranth, rinsed in fine strainer and drained
1 Tbsp. sea salt
6 cups water
Kernels from 8 ears of corn, or 16 oz. frozen corn
1 large onion, minced
1 large red bell pepper, diced
1 mild green chili pepper, diced (optional)
1 tsp. Herbamare
13/4 tsp. Frontier Herbs Mexican Seasoning (salt free)
1/2 tsp. ground cumin

1. In bottom of large stockpot, sauté onion, green chili pepper, Mexican Seasoning, and cumin in oil, ghee, or butter with sea salt until onion is translucent.
2. Add millet, amaranth, corn, and water.
3. Bring water to a boil, cover, turn heat on low, and let cook 30 minutes.
4. Fold in red pepper and Herbamare; adjust seasonings to taste.
5. Pour into a 9″ by 13″ buttered casserole dish, dotting with butter or ghee if desired.
6. Bake 30 minutes at 350 degrees.

Variation: Use 1 Tbsp. Frontier Herbs Italian Seasoning instead of Mexican Blend; and change vegetables to zucchini, shiitake mushrooms, and chopped red bell peppers

To bring out a more delicious corn flavor, make a "stock" by cutting the fresh corn off the cob and simmering the cut corn and the corn cobs in 7 cups of water for 20 minutes. Puree and drain. Use 6 cups of this corn stock in recipe.

Heidi's Savory Crackers—Mexican Variation

Ingredients:
1/2 cup amaranth flour
1/2 cup blue corn flour
1/4 cup arrowroot powder
1/4 tsp. sea salt
1/2 tsp. baking soda
3 Tbsp. softened butter
1/2 tsp. chili powder
1/2 tsp. cumin seed
5 Tbsp. water (approximately)
Herbamare to taste

———

1. Heat oven to 350 degrees.
2. Sift or blend dry ingredients together with a wire whisk.
3. Using a whisk, pastry cutter, or fork, work butter into flour mixture.
4. Add just enough water to make dough stick together to form a ball.
5. On a floured surface, or between wax paper, roll dough flat (approximately 1/4 inch thick).
6. Sprinkle surface lightly with Herbamare.
7. Transfer to greased cookie sheet.
8. Cut into rectangles, squares, triangles, and diamond shapes.
9. Bake for 15 minutes or until edges just begin to brown.
10. Remove from oven and place on wire rack.
11. Place rack of crackers on cookie sheet and put back in oven to become crisp.
12. Turn off oven and serve.

Bill and Mike's Waffles

Waffles, like any flour food, should be an occasional meal. They go nicely with vegetable soup at any time of the day. We have even used them to make sandwiches. We make ours with B.E.D. mayonnaise and a variety of roasted or grilled veggies. These waffles can be frozen or kept for several days in the refrigerator.

(Makes four 9-inch square waffles, which break into smaller squares that fit into a toaster for reheating.)

Ingredients:
2 cups flour (amaranth, half amaranth and half millet, or other grain flour combinations)
1/2 tsp. sea salt
1/4 cup melted butter (1/2 stick)
2 tsp. baking powder (aluminum free)
2 eggs (whites and yolks in two separate bowls)
1–1 1/3 cups water (depends on flour used)

———

1. Preheat waffle iron to medium or dark setting (a little experimentation will determine which is best).
2. Combine flour, sea salt, and baking powder in mixing bowl.
3. Use whisk to thoroughly mix dry ingredients.
4. In separate bowl, combine egg yolks, water, and melted butter; whisk together until barely blended.
5. Add liquid ingredients to dry and whisk together until a smooth batter is formed. (You may need to add more water to batter to correct the consistency. Batter should pour easily into a waffle iron and spread into all corners—not too thick.)
6. In separate bowl, beat egg whites until they form soft peaks—firm but not dry.
7. Carefully fold egg whites into batter. (Try to fold in completely without stirring too much.)
8. Using a glass or plastic measuring cup (aluminum causes batter to break down), pour about 1 cup of batter evenly into all areas of waffle iron (1 cup for a 9-inch-square iron). Do not use too much; the batter should not overflow.
9. Waffles should cook in 10–14 minutes. If in doubt, wait until steam stops rising from waffle iron before looking. Cook until crisp and brown.
10. Always cool extra waffles on wire rack.

The Body Ecology Diet Sauces

The soups, especially the creamy soups, such as Broccoli with Fresh Fennel and Creamy Dilled Cauliflower, make wonderful sauces. You can jazz up the dilled cauliflower by adding shiitake mushrooms and create a dish that is very similar to Campbell's cream of mushroom soup. This can be used as a base in many recipes . . . even some adaptations of old-time family favorites.

When you make the Carrot-Cauliflower with Tarragon Soup, pull out a few cups of soup just after you have blended it, and add a tablespoon (or even more) of whole-grain mustard (made with apple cider vinegar). You now have a delicious new sauce. I (Heidi) steam large chunks of vegetables (onions, celery, carrots, potatoes, broccoli) and pour them into a baking dish with this tarragon/mustard carrot sauce over the top. I bake my vegetable casserole for about 30 minutes. It is absolutely delicious.

The Body Ecology Diet Gravy

This delicious recipe is greatly enhanced by the addition of sautéed onions and shiitake mushrooms. It's great for special

THE BODY ECOLOGY DIET

occasions, such as Thanksgiving and other holidays, when a traditional gravy is needed.

Ingredients:
2 Tbsp. organic, unrefined coconut oil, butter, or ghee
2 1/2–3 Tbsp. amaranth flour
2 cups vegetable broth or water
1/4 tsp. fresh minced garlic
1 tsp. of any one of Spice Hunter's many seasoning blends, such as Herbes de Provence or Deliciously Dill
Sea salt, Trocomare, or Herbamare to taste

———

1. In a small skillet, make a roux by melting ghee, butter or oil and quickly stirring in flour.
2. Very slowly add vegetable broth or water, stirring constantly.
3. Add garlic and seasoning; adjust to taste.

Variation: Sauté sliced onions and shiitake mushrooms in the same skillet you will be using to make the gravy. Remove them and make gravy. Fold onions and shiitakes back in and reheat before serving.

Curried Cauliflower Sauce

Great on millet.

Ingredients:
1–2 Tbsp. organic, unrefined coconut oil, ghee, or butter
1 large onion, chopped
2 cloves garlic, minced
1 1/2 tsp. ginger root, grated
1 Tbsp. curry powder or to taste
1/4 tsp. cayenne
1 head of cauliflower, chopped
1 cup water
Sea salt, Herbamare, or Trocomare to taste
Lemon juice to taste

———

1. Sauté onion, garlic, ginger root, curry powder, and cayenne in oil, ghee, or butter.
2. Add cauliflower and water.
3. Simmer or pressure-cook until tender.
4. Add sea salt and lemon juice.

Easy Bernaise Sauce

Ingredients:
1 egg
1 tsp. raw, organic apple cider vinegar
1 tsp. mustard
1 Tbsp. lemon juice
1/2 cup butter (1 stick)
Sea salt to taste (1/2–1 tsp.)

—⁓—

1. In a blender, combine all ingredients except butter.
2. In a small pot, melt butter.
3. Add melted butter very gradually to blended mixture and serve.

Gingery Carrot Sauce

Great over grains; serves 4 people.

Ingredients:
1 Tbsp. organic, unrefined coconut oil, ghee, or butter
20–25 small carrots, chopped (or 15 large)
2 large onions, diced
3 cloves garlic, minced
2 1/2 stalks celery, chopped
1 small red pepper, chopped
Water or stock to cover
2 1/2 tsp. sea salt or Herbamare
1 Tbsp. Italian seasoning
2 tsp. garlic powder
Ginger juice to taste*

—⁓—

1. Sauté carrots and onions in oil, ghee, or butter.
2. Add celery and red pepper and continue to sauté until tender.
3. Add water and sea salt.
4. Pressure-cook 15 minutes or simmer until very soft.
5. Puree.
6. Add seasonings, ginger juice, and enough water to create the right consistency for a sauce.
7. Stir, and simmer 10–15 minutes.
8. Adjust seasonings.

Variation: Add a pinch of cumin, coriander, or cardamom to carrots as they sauté.

*To make ginger juice: grate ginger, pick up by handful, and squeeze the juice into small measuring cup.

Mock Tomato Sauce

The beet in this recipe is added merely for color and will not cause a problem. This recipe is included for those who love tomato sauces. Adding apple cider vinegar at the end of cooking will more closely duplicate the acidic quality in a tomato sauce. Great over millet or buckwheat croquettes.

Ingredients:
3 Tbsp. organic, unrefined coconut oil, ghee, or butter
4 cups diced red onion
3 Tbsp. garlic, finely chopped
3 Tbsp. pizza seasoning (Spice Hunter)
1 medium zucchini, diced
2 butternut squash
3 cups beet stock*
2 Tbsp. of sea salt
6 cups water
1 cup apple cider vinegar

—◁〰▷—

1. Sauté onions and garlic in oil, ghee, or butter until golden.
2. Add pizza seasoning and zucchini and continue to sauté.

3. Take off heat.
4. Preheat oven to 350 degrees.
5. Poke holes in squash to prevent it from exploding.
6. Bake squash until very soft, approximately 1 1/2–2
    hours.
7. When done, slice in half and let cool enough to handle.
8. Scoop seeds and measure 7 cups of squash meat.
9. Add to mixture of onions and zucchini.
10. Add water and bring up to temperature.
11. Add beet stock.
12. Continue to simmer and puree until smooth.
13. Add water and salt for desired thickness and flavor.
14. When room temperature, add apple cider vinegar.

*Beet stock is made by simmering 1–2 sliced beets in 2 cups
of water for 30 minutes.

Luscious Lemon Butter Sauce

Good poured on an all-vegetable platter.

Ingredients: (makes approximately 2 cups)
1/2 cup butter (1 stick) or ghee
1 Tbsp. organic, unrefined oil
2 medium onions, finely chopped, or 2 small scallions,
    thinly sliced
1/3 cup fresh lemon juice
1/2 heaping tsp. dried tarragon or 1 heaping Tbsp. finely
    torn fresh tarragon
1/2 heaping tsp. dried basil or 1 heaping Tbsp. finely
    chopped fresh basil

1. Heat butter or ghee and oil in a small skillet.
2. Add onions, and sauté until soft.
3. Add remaining ingredients, and simmer 10 minutes.
4. Remove from heat and serve.

Variation: Use 1/2 heaping tsp. dried dill or 1 Tbsp. fresh
dill instead of tarragon and basil.

Pesto

Ingredients:
3–4 cups fresh basil
3/4 cup organic, unrefined flax or pumpkin seed oil*
1 tsp. sea salt
Zest of 1 lemon
3 Tbsp. lemon juice (approximately 1 juicy lemon)
3–4 cloves garlic
1/2 cup flat-leaf parsley
1 Tbsp. lecithin

—⁓—

1. In a blender, combine ingredients.
2. Blend until thoroughly pureed.
3. Serve over noodles, grains, red potatoes, a salad, or a
   platter of vegetables.

*At the time when you are able to introduce olive oil into your diet, it can be used in this recipe in place of the unrefined oil.

The Body Ecology Diet Salads and Salad Dressings

Salads are special foods, and the Body Ecology Diet salads are even more so. Salads can be a meal in themselves . . . they can be made with raw or with cooked and chilled ingredients . . . they're simple to prepare . . . they adhere easily to food-combining rules . . . and they are an important part of a health-building diet.

Although raw foods may be difficult for you to digest, especially when you first start The Diet, they are so rich in enzymes, vitamins, and minerals that it's important for you to include a properly prepared salad in your meals at least once a day as soon as you are able. For easier digestion, try salads with parboiled vegetables and a no-oil dressing (more about this later).

On hot summer days, crisp, cool salads are ideal meals or even snacks. Around the year, you can easily carry them to work and even carry the dressing separately to add at the last moment. When your body becomes contracted from too much salt or a stressful day, balance it with an expansive salad. If your body is too acidic, an alkaline salad can come to the rescue.

Need some salad ideas? See our recipes—and consider the great variety of available lettuces and land, ocean, and cultured vegetables. The more color, the better: green broccoli; asparagus; English peas; yellow squash; red pepper or onion; cool white cucumber or jicama. You can make grain salads with the four B.E.D. grains and potatoes, or protein salads with chopped salmon, tuna, chicken, or turkey. Or mix some soaked almonds, sunflower, or pumpkin seeds in with those veggie salads for extra crunch.

Please don't forget those very special ocean vegetables. Leftover hijiki with onions and carrots (see ocean vegetable recipes starting on page 322) is delicious when tossed with leafy lettuce and radicchio and topped with the Body Ecology Diet Salad Dressing. Or soak some arame in water for ten minutes, drain, and chop; and add it to your green leafy salad. Wakame is delicious in a cucumber salad with diced red pepper and red onion. Cut sheets of nori into small strips or squares to sprinkle on any salad for a color and taste bonus.

Raw cultured vegetables add color and zest to any salad. We even add them to our dressing recipes and to mayonnaise.

Importance of Organic, Unrefined Oils

We used to think that "cold-pressed" or "expeller-pressed" oils sold in health-food stores were healthy. But I (Donna) started working with an enzyme therapist who tested urine samples and found that people simply were not digesting these fats. The problem sent me on an intensive search for an answer. I learned that the liver, a key digestive organ, must have totally unrefined oils. It just wasn't created to process the man-made, refined oils that Americans have been eating for generations. Even if you find them in a health-food store and even if they are labeled "cold-pressed," they are still bleached, deodorized, and refined. They lack essential fatty acids, color, and flavor. Organic, unrefined oils, however, provide you with essntial fatty acids.

You may have noticed that when you eat oils, you become bloated and have gas in your intestines. If so, try keeping all fats and oils to a minimum until your inner ecosystem is established. (See our recipes for oil-free salad dressings.) Beneficial microflora play an important role in digesting fats and oils, so as you begin to eat and drink fermented foods and liquids, this problem may totally disappear. Since fats are digested in your small intestine, you will definitely notice an improvement in your digestion of them if you take a pancreatic enzyme. (Body Ecology offers one called ASSIST SI.) Our goal is to help you create a thriving inner ecosystem so that you can eat and enjoy oils that really are essential for creating ideal health.

Organic, unrefined seed oils are raw and cold-pressed. They are processed with an amazing amount of care. Organic seeds such as flax, pumpkin, evening primrose, borage, rapeseed, sunflower, or safflower are gently pressed to release their oil. The oil is never exposed to light or oxygen, and no preservatives are used. They are packaged in light-proof bottles and are stamped with an expiration date. Since they are stronger and more flavorful than the oils you grew up eating, they may take some getting used to. But most people love the rich taste of these precious oils and would never go back to refined, "plasticized" oils after they learn about the medicinal benefits of unrefined oils.

Flax seed oil is an excellent source of omega-3 fatty acid. We tend to be very deficient in this fatty acid today. Omega-3 is easily destroyed by heat, so we never cook with it on The Diet. Unrefined canola oil (made from rapeseed) is another source of omega-3s but is not used on the B.E.D. because of its strong, bitter flavor. The commercial canola oil you see everywhere these days has no color or flavor, so you know it is refined.

Extra-virgin olive oil enjoys high praise among nutritionists, and many people report they digest it well. Why? It's unrefined. Many stores sell high-quality extra-virgin unrefined olive oil. Olive oil has only trace amounts of essential fatty acids, but it has properties that help protect your heart. You can use it generously on the Body Ecology Diet.

Organic, Raw, Unfiltered Apple Cider Vinegar

People are often surprised to learn they can eat vinegar on the Body Ecology Diet. It's true you can, but only if it is raw, unfiltered apple cider vinegar that has been aged in wood barrels. Several companies make apple cider vinegar, and you will find a nice selection in your health-food store.

Some apple cider vinegars are treated during fermentation with meta-bisulfite, a preservative that is not required by law to be listed on the label. Look for a vinegar that contains natural sediment with pectin, trace minerals, beneficial bacteria, and enzymes. Light causes free-radical activity and a breakdown of vital nutrients. Vinegar packaged in clear glass bottles is vulnerable to oxidation, causing it to turn a brown color.

Thanks to vinegar's mineral content (especially potassium), it has the ability to normalize the body's acid/alkaline balance. Its antiseptic qualities cleanse the digestive tract. The acidity aids in the removal of calcium deposits from joints and blood vessels but has no effect on normal calcium levels of the bones or teeth. Pectin in unfiltered apple cider vinegar promotes elimination and healthy bowels. The potassium in the vinegar regulates growth, hydrates cells, balances sodium, and enables proper performance of the nervous system.

No-Oil Dressings for Better Digestion

Without a healthy inner ecosystem, many people have trouble digesting fats and oils. Furthermore, there are times when you may want or need to avoid oils but still want to enjoy fresh salads with your meals. These times include the following:

1. You're just beginning the B.E.D., and your digestion is not yet strong enough to handle oils. Soon, however, you will be able to easily absorb all the nutrients that the good fats and oils bring.

2. You're giving your liver and gallbladder a rest with a cleansing program that eliminates oils.

Both these situations call for a no-oil dressing. You've probably seen such dressings in stores, but you may not know how to make one. We'll show you how, with a gel fiber called xanthan gum.[24] Simply remove the oil from any favorite dressing recipe, substitute an equal amount of water and a little xanthan gum to thicken, and add a variety of herbs and seasonings. Once you become familiar with xanthan gum, you'll soon be creating dressings of your own. Our recipes are simply guidelines to stimulate your own creativity.

These dressings can be very handy when you want to have a protein meal and a salad. Remember that large amounts of oil (as in a tuna-fish salad with mayo) inhibit the secretion of hydrochloric acid (HCl) in the stomach. You need both HCl and pepsin to digest protein. A tuna-fish salad made with a no-oil or low-oil dressing can taste fabulous. Now you can create egg-, tuna-, and chicken-salad masterpieces, or make an almond, pumpkin seed, or sunflower seed paté, with one of our no-oil recipes.

No-oil dressings and dressings made with only the highest-quality unrefined oils are beginning to play a key role in helping us become healthier. As more of us learn how critical it is to eliminate poor-quality fats and bad cholesterol from our diets, many of the diseases we suffer from today will simply go away.

∼

Notes

[24] Xanthan gum is produced by the pure culture fermentation of the microorganism *Xanthomonas campestris*. It is 100% pure and contains no sugar, salt, starch, yeast, wheat, corn, soy, or milk; it seems to be tolerated by even the most sensitive people. Available from NOW Foods (800-999-8069) and Bob's Red Mill Natural Foods, Milwaukie, Oregon 97222 (800-349-2173). Please tell your health-food store to order it for you.

Salad and Salad Dressing Recipes

Compared to cultured or steamed vegetables, raw vegetables are usually difficult to digest until your inner ecosystem is well established. They are, however, rich in necessary enzymes, and we have found that, properly prepared, a salad once a day is an important part of the Body Ecology Diet. Preparation suggestions in parentheses make these vegetables easier to digest.

The Body Ecology Diet Salad

Choose from among these vegetable greens to create an infinite number of delectable salad combinations:

Beet tops	Lamb's-quarters
Cabbage	Lettuce
Chard	Parsley
Comfrey	Radish tops
Dandelion	Spinach
Endive	Turnip tops
Escarole	Watercress
Kale	

Sprouts that can be added include:
Alfalfa
Radish
Sunflower

Stems and roots:

Broccoli (steamed)	Jerusalem artichokes (shredded)
Carrots (shredded)	Jicama (shredded)
Cauliflower (steamed)	Summer squash
Celery	Zucchini
Corn (blanched)	

Especially nutritious additions:

Arame (soaked or cooked)	Nori (shredded)
Red onions	Chives
Scallions	Hijiki (cooked)
Wakame (soaked)	

Seed and herb seasoning suggestions:

Basil	Dill	Paprika
Cardamom	Garlic Powder	Parsley
Caraway	Horseradish	Poppy Seed
Cayenne	Marjoram	Pumpkin Seed
Celery	Nutmeg	Sage
Cinnamon	Onion Powder	Thyme

The Body Ecology Diet Salad Dressing with Apple Cider Vinegar

To make a portion that serves 1–2 people:

Ingredients:
2 Tbsp. extra-virgin olive oil
1 Tbsp. flax seed oil or a flax seed/evening primrose oil
blend
1 Tbsp. raw, organic apple cider vinegar
(lemon juice is also delicious)
1/4–1/2 tsp. Celtic sea salt and/or Herbamare to taste

More great options: 1–2 tsp. roasted pumpkin seed oil, 1 tsp. mustard, 1 Tbsp. Sea Seasonings Dulse or Dulse with Garlic, dash of homemade mayonnaise (or use Follow Your Heart Vegenaise, made with grapeseed oil), pinch of cayenne, 1/2 tsp. EcoBloom (a prebiotic that encourages the growth of friendly microorganisms)

To make this dressing quickly, place all ingredients into the bottom of a wooden, glass, or stainless-steel salad bowl. Using a wire whisk, quickly whip together all ingredients. Place your favorite salad greens including a variety of lettuces, and fresh herbs (basil, cilantro, arugula) into the bowl and toss thoroughly. Keep tossing until all greens glisten with the dressings. Adjust taste, adding more Celtic sea salt or Herbamare if desired.

Other great additions: Soaked and chopped arame (ocean vegetable), leftover lightly steamed veggies, soaked nuts and seeds, and Kefir cheese (for stage two of the B.E.D.). Kefir cheese is delicious tossed into the B.E.D. Salad Dressing and combines with all raw veggies, cultusred veggies, nuts, and seeds.

To make a larger portion to keep refrigerated:

Ingredients:
2/3 cup organic, unrefined oils (use a combination of
    extra-virgin olive oil, flax seed oil, or a flaxseed/
    evening primrose oil blend)
1/3 cup organic apple cider vinegar (or lemon juice)
1 tsp. Celtic sea salt or to taste
(Add other options from preceding page)

To make this dressing quickly, place all ingredients in a container with a lid and shake vigorously.

To prepare an even creamier version, place the apple cider vinegar and the seasonings in a blender. Blend at medium speed, slowly adding the oil. This "emulsifies" or thickens the salad dressing, and it will not separate. For a thicker dressing, slowly add xanthan gum after oil, and blend. The Cuisinart Quick Prep or other hand-held blenders work well, too. Keep refrigerated for a week to 10 days.

Parboiled Salad

Ingredients:
Variety of lettuce, torn into bite-size pieces
Vegetables to chop for parboiling:

Broccoli	Daikon	String beans
Cabbage	Kale	Yellow squash
Carrots	Peas	Zucchini
Corn (cut off cob)	Radishes	Celery
Scallions	Cucumbers	Red onions

—⁊⁊⁊—

1. Cut various vegetables into pretty shapes (matchsticks, half moons, flowers, stars), using vegetable cutters if you wish.
2. Quickly parboil in rapidly boiling water. Make sure you don't overcook. They are best when taken out of the water right after they have turned their brightest color (e.g., broccoli turns a beautiful bright green).
3. Remove from heat and chill well.

4. In a bowl, place lettuce and chilled vegetables.
5. Toss with a salad dressing of your choice.

Fresh herbs are great, too (chop and add raw): parsley, dill, mint, basil, watercress, arugula.

Ocean vegetables are wonderful: dulse, wakame, arame. Just soak until soft, drain, squeeze out extra liquid, and chop. (You don't have to cook wakame or arame, but you can do so for 15 minutes if desired.)

Soaked and sprouted almonds and raw sunflower seeds add a nice festive touch, but do not add them if your salad has a starchy vegetable like red potatoes.

Salads Using Grain-like Seeds

Remember that on the Body Ecology Diet only four "grains" (really seeds that are grain-like) can be eaten initially. With time you may be able to introduce true grains back into your diet. This recipe works well for millet, quinoa, buckwheat or a combination of the three grains. Later it works well with rice, bulgur, barley, etc. Amaranth is too sticky for a grain salad.

Leftover cooked grains or grain-like seeds can be converted easily into a grain salad since they are usually drier than freshly cooked grain.

When cooking fresh grain to use in your grain salads, bring the water to a boil before you add the grain. Once the grain is cooked, remove it from the heat and let it sit for 15 minutes or longer to dry out and become fluffier.

Toss together 2–4 cups of any cooked grain (or grain combination) with raw or slightly blanched vegetables, add a dressing of your choice, sprinkle in some seasonings or sea salt . . . and your grain salad is complete.

Vegetables should be diced or finely chopped, and ocean vegetables (which make an excellent addition to a creative grain salad) should be soaked or cooked (see Chapter 12).

Vegetable suggestions:

Carrots	Scallions	Yellow squash
Cucumbers	Radishes	Green beans
Celery	Peas	Broccoli
Red onions	Corn	Ocean vegetables

Quinoa Salad

Ingredients:
2 cups uncooked quinoa (or millet)
2/3 cup frozen peas
2/3 cup frozen or fresh corn
2/3 cup red bell peppers, finely diced
1 bunch scallions or 1 red onion, finely chopped (optional)
1 cup or more Rosemary Vinaigrette Dressing (see recipe)

———

1. Cook grain until done but still slightly resilient.
2. Steam carrots, peas, and corn 4–6 minutes (should be cooked but still slightly firm)
3. In a large bowl, combine all ingredients.

Quinoa Tabouli

Ingredients: (serves 4)
1 cup quinoa
2 cups water
1/2 tsp. sea salt
1 cup cucumber, diced small
1/2 cup parsley, finely chopped
1/2 cup scallions, finely sliced
1 cup Mint-Garlic Dressing (see recipe)
Lettuce leaves as a garnish

———

1. Cook quinoa and sea salt in 2 cups of boiling water, until translucent; remove from heat and let sit 10–15 minutes to become fluffy.
2. When cool, add cucumber, parsley, and scallions.
3. Add Mint-Garlic Dressing.
3. Chill in refrigerator before serving.
4. Serve on lettuce leaves.

Celery Root Salad

Ingredients:
Celery root, grated in food processor
Homemade mayonnaise
Pinch of sea salt
Herbs to taste

—◦◦◦—

Combine all ingredients in a salad bowl and serve.

New Red Potato Salad in Red Onion Dressing

Ingredients: (makes 6 servings)
2 lbs. small red potatoes, washed and scrubbed well
Sea salt or Herbamare to taste
Freshly ground black pepper
3/4 cup homemade mayonnaise
1/2 cup sweet red onion, finely chopped
1/2 cup dill, fennel, or parsley, preferably flat-leaf type,
    minced
Fresh dill or parsley sprigs for garnish

—◦◦◦—

1. Cut potatoes into bite-size cubes and cook until tender.
2. When cool, add other ingredients.
3. Chill before serving.

Variations:
Add watercress, mustard, and 1–2 Tbsp. raw, organic apple cider vinegar or herbs such as curry powder, garlic, Italian seasonings, etc. Toss in several spoonfuls of your favorite cultured veggie blend to give this salad even more pizzaz—and, of course, make it more digestible, too.

These same ingredients can be tossed with the Body Ecology Diet Salad Dressing instead of the mayonnaise, and it's even healthier.

Marinated Corn Salad

Ingredients: (makes 4-6 servings)
l 3/4 cups yellow corn, cut from cob (about 4 ears)
1/4 cup water
1/2 small red pepper, cut into 1/2-inch strips
1/2 cup celery, chopped
2 Tbsp. green onions, thinly sliced
1 Tbsp. pimiento, chopped
1 Tbsp. fresh parsley, chopped
3 Tbsp. organic, unrefined flax or pumpkin seed oil
1 Tbsp. raw, organic apple cider vinegar
Sea salt and pepper to taste

———

1. Combine corn and water in a medium saucepan.
2. Bring to a boil; cover, reduce heat, and simmer 7–8 minutes or until corn is tender.
3. Drain corn and combine with red pepper and next 4 ingredients and set aside.
4. Combine oil and remaining ingredients in a jar; cover tightly and shake vigorously.
5. Combine marinade and corn mixture; cover and chill at least 4 hours before serving.

Summertime Curried Corn Salad

For special occasions.

Ingredients:
6–8 ears fresh corn or 3 cups frozen
1 small zucchini, diced
1 large red bell pepper, diced
1 bunch scallions, white and tender part of green, cut into 1/4-inch pieces
1/2 cup Italian parsley, chopped

———

Dressing:
1/4 cup organic, unrefined flax or pumpkin seed oil
4 Tbsp. raw, organic apple cider vinegar or lemon juice

1 tsp. curry powder
1/2 tsp. sea salt
1–2 cloves garlic, minced

1. You can use the corn raw or, if you prefer, blanch it quickly and cool.
2. Combine the raw or cooled corn, zucchini, pepper, scallions, and parsley.
3. Combine the oil, vinegar or lemon juice, curry powder, sea salt and garlic.
4. Combine the vegetables and dressing and marinate 2–4 hours.

Variation: Add 1–2 Tbsp. homemade mayonnaise for a creamier dressing.

Carrot Salad

This salad is excellent for helping eliminate toxins in the colon.

Ingredients: (serves 1–2)
2 Tbsp. organic, unrefined coconut oil
1 Tbsp. organic, unrefined olive oil
4–6 large carrots, peeled and trimmed

Finely grate the carrots in food processor and toss with both oils.

Cole Slaw

Ingredients: (serves 4)
1 small head white cabbage
2 cups boiling water
3 grated carrots
Sea salt to taste
Seasoned mayonnaise or B.E.D. Salad Dressing

1. Cut the cabbage in chunks and grate in food processor or by hand.
2. Place cabbage and carrots into a large mixing bowl and wilt by pouring the boiling water with sea salt over them (this makes for easier digestion). Stir several times and drain.
3. Toss with seasoned mayonnaise or the B.E.D. Salad Dressing.

Variations: Other ingredients can be added such as scallions, red pepper, celery, sliced daikon or red radishes, dill, caraway or celery seed, sunflower seeds, chopped parsley, chives, dill, fennel, or other fresh herbs.

For a sweet cole slaw, add a few drops of stevia concentrate.

Asparagus, Green Beans, and Artichoke Salad

This elegantly arranged salad can stand alone or as a part of an alkaline-forming, all-vegetable meal. It is also delightful with a grain entree. Artichokes are a starchy vegetable, so remember not to serve this salad with animal protein.

Ingredients: (serves 6)
1 lb. cooked asparagus spears, fresh
1/2 lb. green beans, fresh
6 small cooked fresh artichokes or frozen artichoke hearts (see cooking directions on next page)
1/2 cucumber, peeled and thinly sliced
1 red bell pepper, cut into thin strips
1/2 head cauliflower, broken into small florets and steamed lightly or quickly blanched and held under cold water to stop the cooking
1/2 cup organic, unrefined oil
1/4 cup raw, organic apple cider vinegar
Salt and pepper to taste
1 level Tbsp. dried basil or to taste
1 fresh lemon (if cooking artichoke)

1. Toss all the vegetables together in a salad bowl.
2. In a screw-top jar, put oil, vinegar, salt, pepper, and basil. Shake well to combine.
3. Pour the mixture over the salad and toss gently but well; chill.
4. Toss again lightly. Serve from the bowl; or transfer to a platter lined with thinly sliced cucumbers, and arrange tossed salad ingredients in center of platter. Top with artichokes.

To cook the artichoke:
1. Cut off base so it is flush flat, and snap off the small bottom leaves. Cut about 1 inch off the top of the artichoke.
2. Trim off the outer leaves with scissors to form a nice round shape.
3. With both thumbs, open the artichoke from the middle to expose the choke inside. Use a teaspoon to scrape out all of the hairy choke, and push the artichoke back into shape. Brush with lemon juice to prevent it from discoloring and boil in salted water for 15 minutes. Drain and leave to cool before using.

Green Bean Salad

Ingredients:
1 lb. green string beans
2 Tbsp. organic, unrefined oil
1 tsp. raw, organic apple cider vinegar
Salt and pepper to taste
1 small shallot or 3–4 scallions, finely chopped
1 tsp. dried tarragon, oregano, dill, or garlic (optional)
1 sprig of parsley

1. Cut the washed beans into 1-inch lengths and blanch or lightly steam. Drain and rinse with cold water and let cool.
2. Combine oil, vinegar, salt, and pepper in a salad bowl, whisking together well, and add the chopped shallot or scallions.

3. Add the cooled beans and toss together gently. Leave to marinate in refrigerator for an hour.

4. Toss again before serving and garnish with parsley.

No-Oil Salad Dressings

Jeannine's Italian Dressing

Ingredients:

1/2 cup raw, organic apple cider vinegar
1/2 cup freshly squeezed lemon juice
1 1/2 cups water
2 Tbsp. minced garlic
2 Tbsp. whole-grain mustard made with apple cider vinegar
2 Tbsp. finely chopped fresh parsley
2 tsp. sea salt
1/8 tsp. pepper
2 Tbsp. red pepper, finely chopped
1/4 tsp. each: dried oregano, basil, and thyme*
1 tsp. xanthan gum (thickener)

—⁓—

Blend all ingredients except thickener, then add the xanthan gum; blend or shake well. Refrigerate overnight.

*1 tsp. of Spice Hunter's Italian Seasoning blend can be added instead (see Shopping List).

Lemon Rosemary Garlic Dressing

Ingredients:

1 cup raw, organic apple cider vinegar
1 1/2 cups water
1/2 cup freshly squeezed lemon juice
2 Tbsp. minced garlic
1/2 tsp. pepper
1/2 tsp. celery seed
6 Tbsp. red onion, diced
2 Tbsp. red pepper, diced
1 tsp. dill weed
2 Tbsp. fresh parsley, minced

3 tsp. sea salt

2 Tbsp. dried rosemary, crushed, or 4 Tbsp. fresh
   rosemary, crushed

1 tsp. xanthan gum (thickener)

———

Blend first 12 ingredients, then add xanthan gum; blend
   or shake well. Refrigerate overnight.

Rosemary Vinaigrette Dressing

Ingredients:

1/2 cup raw, organic apple cider vinegar

1/2 cup freshly squeezed lemon juice

1 cup water

4 Tbsp. mustard

1 tsp. freshly ground pepper

1 tsp. rosemary

1/2 tsp. sea salt

1 tsp. xanthan gum (thickener)

———

Blend first 7 ingredients, then add xanthan gum; blend
or shake well. Refrigerate overnight. This dressing is great on
potato salad.

Salad Dressings with Organic, Unrefined Oil

Rosemary Vinaigrette Dressing

Ingredients:

1 tsp. rosemary

1/4 cup organic, unrefined oil

3/4 cup water

1/2 cup raw, organic apple cider vinegar

1/2 cup freshly squeezed lemon juice

4 Tbsp. mustard

1 tsp. freshly ground pepper
Sea salt to taste
1/2 tsp. xanthan gum (thickener)

---

1. In a jar with a tight-fitting lid, combine first 8
   ingredients and shake well. Add xanthan gum and
   shake well.
2. Chill before serving. (Dressing keeps up to a week.)

Watercress Dressing

Ingredients:
2 Tbsp. fresh lemon juice
1 Tbsp. raw, organic apple cider vinegar
1/2 tsp. dried tarragon
1/4 cup organic, unrefined oil
Salt and pepper to taste
1 bunch watercress, finely chopped

---

1. Mix together the lemon juice, vinegar, tarragon, oil, salt
   and pepper until well blended.
2. Then stir in the finely chopped watercress.

Mint-Garlic Dressing

Good with Quinoa Tabouli (see recipe).

Ingredients:
1/4–1/3 cup fresh lemon juice, to taste (start with less)
1/2 cup organic, unrefined oil
1–2 cloves garlic, minced (or to taste)
1 Tbsp. fresh mint leaves, minced

---

1. Combine lemon juice, mint, and garlic in a blender.
2. Slowly add oil while blending to emulsify.

Italian Dressing

Ingredients: (yields 11/4 cups)
1 cup organic, unrefined oil
1/2 cup raw, organic apple cider vinegar
1 tsp. sea salt or to taste
1/8 tsp. white pepper
1/2 tsp. dry mustard
2 tsp. Italian-blend seasoning
1 clove garlic, minced

—∞—

1. Combine all ingredients in a jar; cover tightly and shake vigorously.
2. Adjust seasonings to taste.
3. Chill thoroughly.

Variation: Use fresh lemon juice in place of apple cider vinegar.

Mayonnaise

Ingredients:
2 egg yolks (free range)
2 Tbsp. raw, organic apple cider vinegar
1 Tbsp. fresh lemon juice
1/2 tsp. mustard
1/8 tsp. cayenne pepper
2 tsp. sea salt or to taste
1 cup olive oil, or 1/2 cup olive and 1/2 cup unrefined safflower oil

—∞—

1. In blender, combine egg yolks, vinegar, lemon juice, mustard, cayenne pepper, salt, and 1/4 cup oil.
2. Blend for 30 seconds.
3. With blender running low, remove insert top and drizzle remaining oil in a thin stream until mixture is thick.
4. Scrape into a glass jar with a screw top, and it will keep safely in your refrigerator 7–14 days.

Variations:

1. Add garlic powder, a dash of white pepper, 1/4 tsp. mustard powder, and herbs (chervil, tarragon, dill, oregano, basil, cumin, coriander, curry, paprika).

2. Cayenne and/or lime juice gives the mayonnaise a nice flavor for topping aspics or for mixing into any salads made of lightly steamed and chilled vegetables such as carrots, broccoli, cauliflower, daikon, kohlrabi, celery root, etc.

3. Mayonnaise can be sweetened with a few drops of stevia liquid concentrate, if desired.

4. In place of the vinegar, add 2 tsp. lemon peel, finely grated, 2 tsp. fresh lemon juice, and 1 tsp. fresh mustard.

Almond Mayonnaise

This recipe is adapted from *The American Vegetarian Cookbook*, a masterpiece by Marilyn Diamond, co-founder of the Fit For Life movement. While Marilyn has included it in her book as an alternative to mayonnaise made with eggs, we think it makes an excellent party dip or snack food when served with raw vegetables.

Ingredients: (yields 11/2–2 cups)
1/2 cup raw almonds
1/2–3/4 cup water
1/4 tsp. garlic powder
3/4 tsp. sea salt
1 cup organic, unrefined oil (flax or pumpkin seed)
3 Tbsp. lemon juice
1/2 tsp. raw, organic apple cider vinegar

1. Cover almonds with boiling water; allow to cool slightly. Slip off skins and have all other ingredients ready.
2. Place almonds in blender or food processor and grind to a fine powder. Add half the water along with garlic powder and seasonings. Blend well, then add the remaining water to form a smooth cream.

3. With blender running low, remove insert top and
drizzle the oil in a thin stream until mixture is thick.
4. Keep blender running and add lemon juice and vinegar.
Blend on low 1 minute longer to allow mixture to
thicken to desired consistency.
5. Scrape into a jar with a screw top and refrigerate. This
will keep 10 days–2 weeks.

Note: If you have trouble digesting oil, eliminate it
completely and increase the water.

☙

Introduction to Ocean Vegetables

We say ocean vegetables, and you may think, *Ugh—seaweed.* Or you might think, *I can follow everything on the Body Ecology Diet except this.* Well, we now want to do whatever we can to encourage you to incorporate these great nutritional gifts into your diet at least once or twice a day. Your current state of health, your desire to restore your body ecology, and surviving in an increasingly toxin-laden environment make ocean vegetables one of the most important new foods you will encounter in your lifetime.

Ocean vegetables are important to restoring your body ecology because they naturally control the growth of pathogenic bacteria, fungi, and viruses. A body-ecology imbalance or immune disorder causes a severe mineral deficiency, plus we have been eating foods grown in mineral-deficient soil for most of our lives. Ocean vegetables are rich in minerals and trace elements lacking in our diets today, and these are structured in such a way that the body can utilize them easily. So we digest and assimilate them well, and they are key to restoring and maintaining proper acid/alkaline balance in the body.

With a body-ecology imbalance, the stomach lacks hydrochloric acid and the enzymes needed for digesting protein. Proper assimilation of protein is necessary in order to absorb minerals, so a mineral deficiency develops, even if sufficient minerals are contained in our food. Our mineral needs are as great as our need for oxygen, and an imbalance of minerals can cause problems such as mood swings and muscle paralysis.

Ocean vegetables strengthen the nervous and immune systems, and they actually have the ability to remove radioactive elements, carcinogens, and even environmental pollutants for those of us who are environmentally sensitive or allergic. They can also provide the calcium that we miss by not having dairy products, and they offer large amounts of chlorophyll.

Ocean vegetables (you may also find them called sea vegetables) are really algae colonies or single-cell organisms. They're red, blue, green, and black. They thrive only in clean water and are harvested just like land vegetables, at certain times of the year; then they are sun dried, packaged, and stored. They grow on rocks or other ocean surfaces.

More Benefits

Asian and island people have used ocean vegetables for thousands of years. They call them "beauty foods" because they help prevent aging and enhance and prolong the color of hair and lips. The long, lustrous hair of Asian women is often attributed to a diet rich in ocean vegetables such as black hijiki and arame. In areas of Japan where ocean vegetables are harvested, the women in their 60s who gather them often look as if they are in their 30s.

Native Americans reportedly traveled to the coasts to collect these special edibles, then returned home with a lightweight addition to their food supply. Dulse is so well accepted in Canada's maritime provinces that you will find it alongside the fresh fruits and vegetables in grocery stores. Ocean vegetables such as agar are often used as stabilizers in processed foods, though we're not aware of that because the law does not require that processing aids be listed as ingredients.

People who eat a macrobiotic diet are familiar with ocean vegetables and their amazing regenerative powers. Thanks to the many years of effort by macrobiotic leaders, ocean vegetables are now widely available in this country, and so are many delicious, creative recipes. We've included only three recipes in this section, but we encourage you to take macrobiotic cooking classes or refer to the many macrobiotic cookbooks for recipes. Most of these recipes call for shoyu or tamari, but you can just substitute salt. Mirin, a sweet wine, is often used to counter the salty taste, but don't use that. Long, slow cooking at a very low temperature, using lots of onions and carrots to sweeten, is the more delicious and medicinal way to cook the stronger-flavored ocean vegetables like hijiki and arame.

Ocean vegetables are a rich source of organic compost material for farmers. According to one fascinating report, the Irish transformed a barren, rocky seaside cliff into fertile soil by fertilizing it with ocean vegetables. If you want to see what they can do, try working some into a house plant and watch it grow.

Ocean Vegetables and the Thyroid

With a body-ecology imbalance, the thyroid never functions properly. Thyroid problems can lead to obesity, excessive thinness, hypertension, flatulence, stubborn cases of constipation, fatigue, nervousness, depression, headaches, and neck and shoulder pain. Ocean vegetables have a medicinal and regulating effect upon the thyroid.

A weak thyroid causes weak digestion because of its influence on the liver, gallbladder, pancreas, bile ducts, and colon. As you will remember from the chapter on colon care, cleansing of the colon is vital to restoring your health. Ocean vegetables, high in natural mineral salts, have a *toning* effect on the colon. Constipation is usually a combined problem of the colon, the liver, and the adrenals. Ocean vegetables supply all these organs with the minerals needed for them to function properly.

The thyroid affects your sensory nerves. Within two to three weeks of eating ocean vegetables every day, you will notice a calmness in both mind and body. Ocean vegetables reduce tension, help you cope with stress, and enable your body to store energy.

The thyroid influences the health of the ovaries, the prostate gland, and the pyloris. If you suffer from indigestion, it's especially important to eat ocean vegetables. It's common to have problems with the pylorus, the valve at the end of the stomach that must open and close at the correct time to allow food to pass into the small intestine. Ocean vegetables are an excellent remedy.

Easy Ways to Use Ocean Vegetables

To ensure that you assimilate the precious minerals in your ocean vegetable dishes, be sure to eat protein-rich foods. B.E.D. grains are high in protein, and the ocean vegetables themselves contain more protein and amino acids (the building blocks of protein) than beans. Ocean vegetables combine well with grains, starches, and animal protein.

Dulse can be eaten right from the package as a snack. In the early 1900s, taverns served dulse as a snack, since its saltiness increased patrons' thirst and therefore tavern revenues. Little did they know it also helped balance the effect of the liquor and beer, which leach minerals from the body. Dulse is high in iron. Carry it with you and eat some when you need energy or brain food. It's an important ingredient in our Body Ecology Diet Salad Dressing. I (Donna) sauté thinly sliced onion; then add dulse, a little water, and some sea salt; cover this with a lid; and let it simmer for about 20 minutes for a delicious, quick vegetable to top a leftover grain. Children love dulse, too.

Nori is also popular with children and can be carried as a snack food. When a sheet of nori is filled with a hot B.E.D. grain or animal food, then rolled up, it makes a convenient "sandwich." Nori is used in Japanese restaurants for making sushi. Try toasting it by passing it quickly over a burner until it changes color from black to green; then crumble it or cut it into thin strips; and use these to garnish soups, grain dishes, or salads.

Kombu can be soaked overnight in spring water to create a mineral-rich broth. Use this medicinal stock when making soups or for cooking your grains. If you dry strips of kombu at a low temperature in your oven, they become crispy like bacon and make a great snack.

Agar is used to create delicious aspics, puddings, and gelatin desserts. You'll find it in several recipes in this book: Vanilla Pudding, Sweet Carrot "Gelatin" Salad (see stevia recipes), and Jelled Butternut Squash. It is superior to animal gelatin, lubricates the digestive tract, and has mild laxative properties. The flakes are easy to work with. As a rule of thumb, for every cup of liquid in your recipe, add a heaping tablespoon of agar flakes. For a savory aspic, simmer fish stock with seasonings and diced non-starchy vegetables; chill; and serve.

Agar is fun to work with. If your aspic needs more seasoning or failed to gel properly, you can melt it down in a saucepan, work with it a little more, then gel it again. Always add the agar to cold water, never hot, and cook it about 20 to 30 minutes on a low simmer. It starts to gel at room temperature but firms up faster with refrigeration.

Arame's fine shredded strands have a crisp texture and sweet, nutty flavor. It should be soaked about 15 minutes, chopped, and tossed into a salad without cooking. If you want to cook it, we've included a simple basic recipe using lots of carrots and onions to sweeten it. We often mix arame with onions and carrots into leftover grains, form it into patties, and sauté it in unrefined oil or ghee. Delicious!

Hijiki has a mild and slightly salty or "fishy" flavor. It quadruples in volume when you soak it. It requires more thorough rinsing, longer soaking, and a longer cooking time than the other ocean vegetables. Simmer at least 45 minutes to an hour until it's really tender. Cooked with onions and carrots, as shown in our recipe, it practically melts in your mouth.

Wakame adds a pretty green color and a delicate flavor to soups and salads. Soak it until soft, cut off the tough spine, chop it, and add to any soup or salad of your choice. Our Cucumber, Wakame, and Red Pepper Salad is very popular.

Tips on Preparing and Storing Ocean Vegetables

These foods can be stored for years. Buy them in bulk to save money, and store them in a cool, dry place. Don't seal them tightly in plastic because if any moisture gets into the container, mold will grow. Before you cook them, check ocean vegetables for tiny shells or stones caught in the folds; rinse them briefly before soaking or putting them in the cooking pot.

Even though they come from a salty environment, ocean vegetables are not salty. Like ocean fish, they absorb very little of the ocean's salt, so be sure to use a high-quality sea salt and season lightly, just to taste.

When you soak most ocean vegetables (except kombu and wakame), please don't use the soaking water for cooking. However, your house plants will love it.

Ocean Vegetable Recipes

Cucumber, Wakame, and Red Pepper Salad

Ingredients:
1/2 oz. wakame (1/4 of 2 oz. bag)
4 large cucumbers, peeled and very thinly sliced
2 tsp. Herbamare or sea salt
1 large red pepper, diced
1 small red onion, finely chopped
1/3 cup raw, organic apple cider vinegar
2 Tbsp. organic, unrefined oil
Pinch of pepper

—ᗡᗢ—

1. Soak wakame for 15 minutes, in enough water to cover.
2. Sprinkle Herbamare or sea salt on cucumbers and let set for several minutes to release the juices.
3. Remove stem from wakame and discard the soaking water.
4. Chop wakame and add to cucumbers.
5. Add diced red pepper and red onion to cucumbers and wakame.
6. Toss in vinegar, oil, and pepper.

Jelled Butternut Squash

Ingredients:
3 cups water
5–6 Tbsp. agar flakes
1 small onion, diced into small chunks
4 cups diced butternut squash
1 tsp. Herbamare or sea salt
1/2 tsp. dill weed

1. Place the water and agar flakes in a pot.
2. Bring to a boil, stirring frequently to dissolve the flakes.
3. Add the squash, onion, and Herbamare; reduce heat to medium-low and simmer until tender.
4. Puree until smooth.
5. Add dill.
6. Pour the hot puree into oiled gelatin mold.
7. Refrigerate until jelled.
8. Slice and serve garnished with parsley, thinly sliced red pepper strips, and a dollop of B.E.D. Mayonnaise. A pinch of curry and/or ginger can be added to the mayonnaise. Rosemary Vinaigrette Dressing (see recipe) also makes a nice topping. Toast slivered, sprouted almonds and sprinkle on top.

Variation:
1. For a spicier version, add 1 tsp. curry seasoning (Spice Hunter).

2. Try using carrots, broccoli, or cauliflower in place of squash. Top with your favorite salad dressing.

3. To make a sweet version, use 1 tsp. Frontier Herbs butterscotch alcohol-free extract and stevia liquid concentrate to taste.

Hijiki (or Arame) with Onions and Carrots

Ingredients:
2 oz. bag dry hijiki
1 large onion, diced
2 large carrots, diced
1 tsp. organic, unrefined coconut oil
Sea salt to taste
Water to cover

1. Soak hijiki for 15 minutes.
2. Sauté onion in oil; add carrots.
3. Drain hijiki, dice, and add to onion and carrots.
4. Cover with water and simmer for 45 minutes to an hour, checking occasionally to make sure water has not evaporated.
5. Add sea salt to taste during the last 10 minutes of cooking.

Variation: Add diced red skin potatoes and/or peas.

Note: To create one of our most popular salads, we chill this basic recipe and toss with leafy lettuce and top with B.E.D. Salad Dressing.

Introduction to Stevia

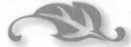

Stevia is an extraordinarily sweet herb. A member of the chrysanthemum family (closely related to tarragon and chamomile and distantly related to lettuce and artichokes), it is totally safe and has been used for centuries by the Guarani Indians of South America, where it grows wild.

The natural stevia plant, which is 200 to 300 times sweeter than sugar, has a strong licorice-like flavor. Over four decades ago, in search of a safe substitute for sugar, the Japanese developed the technology to create an extract of the sweetest elements, stevioside and rebaudioside A, leaving behind most of the licorice-like aftertaste.

I (Donna) brought this white extract powder to the US in 1995 and later developed the liquid concentrate that is even easier to use at home. Most of us with a sweet tooth, and all the children *we* have ever met, love the flavor of stevia liquid concentrate. For some people who only like the taste of real sugar, it may take a little getting used to, but it is well worth learning some simple recipes and new ways to use and enjoy it.

Stevia is almost calorie free, so dieters love it. It is ideal for children, since it allows them to enjoy the sweet taste without the damage of sugar. And today, since most children are born with a yeast infection, it is vital that they not eat sugar in any form right from birth. Moms like knowing that a dessert or beverage made with stevia also helps prevent cavities.

Stevia is a must to help you increase your energy so that you can heal. Unlike sugar, it does not trigger a rise in blood sugar. You won't get a sudden burst of energy followed by fatigue and a need for another "fix." Most important for our purposes, it does not feed yeast or other microorganisms.

Stevia is available in a number of forms, including crushed green leaves and a crude greenish-brown syrup. These two forms have the strong, licorice-like aftertaste. To satisfy our perfectly natural desire for sweet-tasting foods, we prefer using a convenient liquid concentrate, made from a white powder that is low in a component called reb C and high in reb A. This is the secret to why Body Ecology's stevia is so delicious and has no licorice-like aftertaste. To make it, the stevia/reb A blend is extracted from the raw plant using no heat or alcohol. You can find stevia in many health-food stores today, but be aware that there are different strengths available, and you may be disappointed in some brands. Since there is only a very tiny amount of rebaudioside in each leaf of the stevia plant, it is expensive to extract, but it yields the most delicious taste. If you have trouble obtaining high-quality stevia to use in our recipes, call us at 866-4BE-DIET. Your local health-food store can order it from us, too.

If you purchase white powder, we'd like to share an important tip. Since the powder is so potent, at times you may find it difficult to work with and will over-sweeten your foods. That's why we recommend starting to familiarize yourself with stevia by first using the liquid concentrate and experimenting with a few drops at a time to find your own personal level of desired sweetness. Use the powder for cooking or making larger quantities of food.

Stevia is especially delicious with the flavor of fruit and with dairy foods. However, it is not as versatile for baking. Stevia is wonderful in teas and coconut milk and in coconut meat dishes. It's great to sweeten the sour foods like Body Ecology's probiotic beverages (InnergyBiotic, young coconut kefir, and milk kefir.) Use it to sweeten quinoa flakes cooked into a cereal for breakfast.

Baked goods sweetened only with stevia do not rise as high as cakes and muffins baked with sugar, honey, fruit juice, and other popular sweeteners. They also do not brown as much. Check for doneness by touching and not by color. For baking we recommend Lakanto from Japan (**www.bodyecology.com**).

Stevia tastes strong in bland foods, so use much less. It disappears in stronger flavors like carob or chocolate, so use more. Stevia recipe books published by authors unaware of candidiasis combine stevia with various other sweeteners.**

**NOTE: You will find lots more stevia tips in *The Stevia Cookbook: Cooking with Nature's Calorie-Free Sweetener*. But please be advised that I (Donna) wrote this book for mainstream Americans, hoping to teach them about this wonderful alternative to sugar. It contains over 100 recipes using only stevia as a sweetener, but as I mentioned before, many of those recipes (like cheesecake) are not appropriate for anyone fighting a serious immune disorder like candidiasis or cancer.

Visit our stevia website at: Stevia.net

Stevia Recipes

Body Ecology Diet "Acidophilus Milk"

(Many mothers have found that their very young children have enjoyed this "milk" in a bottle. It's a good way to make sure your baby is getting plenty of the friendly microflora, and it satisfies the desire for sugar.)

Ingredients:
1 cup water
1–3 drops B.E.D. stevia liquid concentrate or to taste
1 Tbsp. probiotic powder such as Life Start by Natren
1 tsp. vanilla (non-alcoholic)
1 tsp. lecithin granules (optional)

———

Puree all ingredients in a blender or shake in a jar.

Since dairy does combine with acidic fruits, there is no problem drinking this "milk" and then eating a grapefruit or drinking lemon and water.

Ginger Ale

The ale tastes best when the syrup concentrate is allowed to sit in the refrigerator overnight before using.

Syrup concentrate for the ale:
3 1/2 cups water
4-inch-long piece of ginger, peeled and chopped
2 Tbsp. vanilla flavoring (non-alcoholic)
3 tsp. lemon flavoring (non-alcoholic)
25 drops of stevia liquid concentrate (or to taste)

—◦◦◦—

Serving the ale: (1 cup sparkling mineral water per serving)
1. Boil down ginger in water for 10 minutes.
2. Strain out ginger pieces and pour ginger juice into jar.
3. Add vanilla and lemon flavorings and stevia.
4. Let cool and store in refrigerator as a syrup concentrate.
5. Add 1/8–1/4 cup of syrup to 6–8 oz. of Gerolsteiner Sparkling Mineral Water and serve.

Vanilla Pudding

Ingredients:
4 cups water
1 Tbsp. agar powder or 4 heaping Tbsp. agar flakes
2 Tbsp. arrowroot powder
1/2 tsp. sea salt
1 Tbsp. lecithin granules
2 Tbsp. ghee
1 Tbsp. stevia working solution (1 tsp. white stevia powder dissolved in 3 Tbsp. water)
4 Tbsp. vanilla flavoring
3 small yellow squash, seeds removed, chopped, cooked, drained, and pureed

—◦◦◦—

1. Dissolve agar in 2 cups water.
2. Dissolve arrowroot in 2 Tbsp. water.
3. Combine, and cook on low heat until thickened.

4. Add sea salt, lecithin, ghee, stevia, and remaining water.
5. Simmer 10–15 minutes; pour into baking dish to cool and gel (several hours at room temperature, or faster with refrigeration).
6. When firm, place in blender and blend until smooth.
7. Add pureed yellow squash and vanilla and continue blending until very creamy.

The recipe on this page is not a strict Body Ecology recipe. We offer it as an answer to the many requests for a party recipe that children will eat. With no sugar, wheat, or refined oils, it is a better choice than cookies found in grocery or even health-food stores. You'll be able to enjoy an occasional treat of this quality once you have reestablished your inner ecology and find your digestion is working well.

Look for more sugar-free recipes in *The Stevia Cooking: with Nature's Calorie-Free Sweetener,* by Ray Sahelian, M.D., and Donna Gates.

Norma's Almond Butter Cookies

This recipe is wheat free and gluten free.

Ingredients:
1 stick of unsalted butter, softened
3/4 tsp. Body Ecology's white stevia powder
1 large egg
1 cup almond butter
2 tsp. non-aloholic vanilla flavoring
1/2 tsp. sea salt
1/2 tsp. baking soda
1 1/2 cups Fearn Rice Baking Mix
Cinnamon/Stevia Sprinkles for topping (see recipe on next page)

1. Preheat oven to 350 degrees. Grease a cookie sheet and set aside.
2. In a medium bowl, beat butter with a wire whisk until light and fluffy.
3. Add stevia and cinnamon. Beat until smooth.

4. Beat in egg, almond butter, vanilla flavoring, sea salt, baking soda, and baking mix until blended.
5. Drop cookie dough onto cookie sheet. The dough should be thick enough to hold its shape on a tablespoon.
6. Score cookies by lightly pressing the back of a fork across each one twice in a crisscross pattern.
7. Sprinkle each cookie lightly with Cinammon/Stevia Sprinkles.
8. Bake 15 minutes or until lightly browned.

Cinnamon/Stevia Sprinkles

Tasty over breakfast cereal, cookies, and squash dishes.

Ingredients:
1 tsp. ground cinnamon
1/8 tsp. white stevia powder
Dash of Madagascar Bourbon Vanilla Powder (optional)

———

1. Place ingredients in a small jar or shaker and shake until mixed well.
2. Store with other spices and serve as a garnish.

Sweet Carrot "Gelatin" Salad

This recipe is great for potlucks. If you increase the quantities of ingredients, do not increase the amount of stevia. Always be sure to test for taste.

Ingredients:
3 1/2 cups water
3 medium carrots, shredded
2 stalks celery, finely shredded
1 Tbsp. agar powder (or 4 Tbsp. agar flakes)
1/4 tsp. salt
1/8 tsp. stevia powder
1/2 cup lemon or lime juice (or blend of the two)
Grated rind of 1 lemon

1. In saucepan, dissolve agar powder in 2 cups cold water.
2. Add lemon rind and salt.
3. Bring to a boil, boil 5 minutes.
4. Add celery and boil 1 minute more.
5. Add carrots, stevia, and 1 1/2 cups water; continue boiling 3 minutes more so that carrots are desired tenderness.
6. Mix well.
7. Pour in lemon juice.
8. Pour mixture into mold, bowl, or square baking dish.
9. Serve on bed of lettuce with a dollop of mayonnaise.

Corn Chutney

Ingredients:
1–2 onions, chopped
6 ears corn, kernels removed
3 Tbsp. organic, unrefined oil
1/2 red pepper, diced
1/2 green pepper, diced
9 Tbsp. raw, organic apple cider vinegar
1 tsp. white stevia powder
2–3 cloves garlic, minced
2 Tbsp. grated ginger
3 tsp. chili powder
1/8 tsp. cinnamon
1/8 tsp. ground cloves
1/8 tsp. nutmeg
1/4–1/2 tsp. curry powder
1 Tbsp. arrowroot powder, dissolved in 2 Tbsp. water

1. In a frying pan, sauté onions.
2. Add all additional ingredients except arrowroot.
3. Cook for 5–10 minutes.
4. Add arrowroot dissolved in water.
5. Stir well, simmer for another 3–5 minutes, and serve.

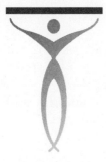

Introduction to Lakanto

The zero-calorie sweetener that looks and tastes like sugar!

Let's face it, there are times when something deliciously sweet would be welcome. Yet, when we do eat it, many of us feel guilty . . .

This desire for sweet-tasting foods and drinks is quite normal. In fact, our very first food, mother's milk, was warm and sweet, and we've formed an emotional bond with this taste.

Avoiding this taste is not the answer!

But as you know, refined white sugar or corn syrup is poison, and even natural sweeteners like agave and honey will feed yeast and make our blood more acidic. So what do we do?

Introducing LAKANTO, the closest natural sweetener to sugar EVER!

Imagine being able to make sweet treats for yourself and your family that actually taste like you used sugar. I (Donna) am thrilled to be able to bring this wonderful new, zero-calorie sweetener to the US.

Is Body Ecology Abandoning Stevia?

NEVER! We fought long and hard to bring stevia to the US market, too . . .

While stevia is perfect for drinks and some recipes, it is not ideal for traditional *baked goods*. And you can't *sprinkle* stevia onto things like you can sugar. Lakanto fills that void.

Lakanto does not feed the harmful yeast (candida) and bacteria in your body. Lakanto is even safe for diabetics!

Lakanto, the amazing all-natural sweetener, has:

- Zero calories
- Zero glycemic index
- Zero additives
- No influence on your blood sugar and insulin release
- A one-to-one ratio with sugar—so it's easy to measure and use

Lakanto is truly part of the next generation of healthy sweeteners.

Lakanto is manufactured in Japan by Saraya Corporation . . . a company with a decades-long history of bringing the finest natural products to the Japanese. Lakanto has been safely enjoyed in Japan for more than years. In fact, over 9,000 hospitals serve Lakanto to their patients.

The Japanese Ministry of Health doesn't just approve Lakanto for use in Japan; they actually recommend it for weight loss, obesity, and blood sugar problems, like diabetes. Lakanto has "generally recognized as safe" (GRAS) status here in the US.

What Is Lakanto Made From?

The two natural ingredients in Lakanto are erythritol (made by fermentation) and the supersweet extract of the luo han guo fruit from China.

Erythritol is a sugar alcohol naturally found in grapes, pears, mushrooms, soy sauce, cheese, wine, and beer, so it has been part of the human diet for thousands of years.

You may be familiar with other sugar alcohols—like xylitol, sorbitol, and maltitol—used in sugar-free candies and chewing gum. But erythritol is different and much better than these other sugar alcohols because it is *fermented*. Yes, it is made by fermenting the sugar in corn. And we sourced out non-genetically modified corn and paid extra to obtain it!

Many people have trouble with foods sweetened with sugar alcohols. Diarrhea, gas, and bloating are frequent complaints. But Lakanto does not cause this problem. We believe it may be because Lakanto is made by this process of fermentation, while the other sugar alcohols are made from hydrogenation.

Because of our high standards at Body Ecology, we asked Saraya Corporation to take one extra step for us. Most erythritol is made from the sugar in genetically modified corn. We asked Saraya to produce the Lakanto that they made for the US market from GMO-free corn. It was costly, but they did this for us.

Erythritol is:

- Specially fermented from non-GMO corn so that you know it's safe.

- Naturally low calorie because your body excretes about 90% of it.

The 10% that remains in your system turns into harmless gases and short-chain fatty acids in your large intestine. (No, Lakanto will not cause embarrassing flatulence.)

Erythritol is sweet, but when used alone in a product, does not taste like sugar. Only when it was combined with the sweet-tasting and medicinal fruit luo han guo . . . in a unique patented process that took two years to develop . . . was Saraya able to create an amazing replica of sugar.

The exotic luo han guo fruit grows high in the Chinese mountains, in the Guangxi province.

The Chinese have been using luo han guo fruit as a sweetener and natural remedy for years. They dry the fruit, which has a sweet toffee or caramel-like flavor, and use it in teas to ease fever, coughing, and phlegm. They even use the tea for digestive troubles.

In fact, the Chinese call luo han guo the "longevity fruit," probably because the people who live where it is cultivated often reach the ripe old age of 100!

Scientists have studied luo han guo and its health benefits extensively, and they've found that this rare fruit has amazing health properties.

Studies have shown that mogrosides (compounds found in the extract of luo han guo) have these properties:

- Anti-carcinogenic
- Regulate blood sugar
- Able to prevent and decrease oxidative stress related to diabetes
- Prevent tooth decay
- Anti-inflammatory
- Inhibit tumor growth
- Antioxidant
- Antihistiminic

Luo han guo extract in Body Ecology's Lakanto has:

- **Zero calories:** Your body does not break down the unique chemical components of the fruit like other simple sugars and carbohydrates.

- **Zero glycemic index:** Because your body metabolizes luo han guo differently, your blood glucose and insulin levels do not rise like they do with other sugars.

- **Zero additives:** Lakanto is made of the natural extract of the luo han guo fruit and erythritol.

When you first taste it right out of the package, you'll notice that Lakanto actually has a flavor that is reminiscent of maple syrup but in a crystal form. It also looks a lot like turbinado sugar, the coarse granulated brown sugar you might have seen in health-food stores, but Lakanto has none of the calories or health risks.

Lakanto looks like sugar, tastes like sugar, bakes like sugar, smells like sugar!

Lakanto Recipes

Wheat- and Gluten-Free Zucchini Bread

Ingredients:
2 cups Pamela's baking mix
1/2 cup Lakanto
2 cups finely shredded zucchini
1/3 cup palm oil (vegetable shortening) by Spectrum
3 eggs
1 1/4 tsp. cinnamon
2 tsp. vanilla
1/2 tsp. salt
Pinch nutmeg
1/2 tsp. lemon zest
3/4 cup chopped walnuts (optional)

1. Preheat the oven 350 degrees. Grease and flour 9″ by 5″ loaf pan.
2. In a large bowl, combine baking mix, Lakanto, cinnamon, salt, and nutmeg. In a separate bowl, combine shortening, vanilla, zucchini, eggs, and lemon zest. Mix wet ingredients into dry; add nuts and fold in.
3. Bake 55–60 minutes or until golden brown or skewer inserted in the center comes out clean. (May take up to 1 1/2 hours in some ovens.)

Teriyaki Sauce

Ingredients:
2/3 cup tamari
4 tsp. Lakanto
2 tsp. vinegar
2 tsp. ginger
2 cloves garlic
1/4 tsp. sea salt
1/4 tsp. xanthan gum

Excellent for grilling, marinades, or basting on meat, poultry, and vegetables.

Green Onion Salad Dressing

Ingredients:
1 cup extra-virgin olive oil
1/2 cup Lakanto
1/4 cup raw, organic apple cider vinegar
1/4 tsp sea salt
1 bunch of green onions (5 or 6)

Put all ingredients in blender and blend until smooth. Will be somewhat thick.

I (Donna) have created a recipe book with more delicious Lakanto recipes. The Lakanto sweetener and the cookbook can be ordered online at: **www.bodyecology.com**.

Appendix A

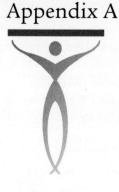

The Body Ecology
Diet Shopping List

Buy organic foods whenever possible.

A sensitivity to any one of the foods in this list, while uncommon, is a *not* uncommon when you have digestive problems and immune deficiency. As you create a healthy inner ecosystem, and strengthen your digestion and immune system, you should soon be able to enjoy most of these foods. But remember the principle of uniqueness. Find foods that work best for your unique body. We have carefully examined the ingredients in the brand names mentioned below and have given them the B.E.D. stamp of approval (Υ). As we learn about new safe and delicious foods and products that help you become even healthier, we will expand and update this list.

ANIMAL PROTEIN
(Free from antibiotics or hormones)
Eggs, from free-range poultry (the best come directly from farmer)
Fish and fish eggs (roe), cold-water, fresh, and frozen
Premium grass-fed ground beef (one supplier we like is White Oak Pastures [Bluffton, GA], available at Whole Foods and Publix Markets)
Free-range poultry
Natural beef and turkey hot dogs and sausage (Applegate Farms: **www.applegatefarms.com**)

———∿∿∿———

BAKING PRODUCTS
Alcohol-free flavoring extracts
(Frontier: **www.frontiercoop.com**; St. John's Botanicals: **www.stjohnsbotanicals.com**; and The Spicery Shoppe)
Baking powder
(Hain Pure Foods: **www.hainpurefoods.com**)
Pure vanilla powder (Nielsen-Massey Vanillas, Inc.: **www.nielsenmassey.com**)

———∿∿∿———

BUTTER/GHEE
(Preferably from grass-fed cows; many grass-feeding farmers advertise butter in *Wise Traditions in Food, Farming, and the Healing Arts*, the journal of the Weston A. Price Foundation)
Body Ecology's **Culture Starter**
(for homemade cultured butter—even raw)
X-Factor Gold High-Vitamin Butter Oil
(Green Pasture Products: **www.greenpasture.org**)
Butter (raw best)
Ghee, also called clarified butter
(Purity Farms is organic: **www.purityfarms.com**)

———∿∿∿———

DAIRY*
(Visit **www.realmilk.com** for sources near you)
Hawthorne Valley Farm raw cow's milk
(NY: **www.hawthornevalleyfarm.org**)

Claravale Farm raw cow's milk
  (CA: **http://claravaledairy.com**)
Organic Pastures raw cow's milk
  (CA: **www.organicpastures.com**)
Sweetwoods Dairy raw goat's milk (NM: 505-465-2608)
Peaceful Pastures raw cow's and goat's milk (TN: **www. peacefulpastures.com**)

—◊◊◊—

ENZYMES

Body Ecology's **Assist™ Full Spectrum Plant Digestive Enzyme Formula** (for vegetarian meals)
Body Ecology's **Assist™ Dairy & Protein**
  (effectively digests animal-protein meals)
Body Ecology's **Assist SI™**
  (digests protein, carbs, and fats in small intestines; use at every meal)

—◊◊◊—

FERMENTED FOODS

Body Ecology has starter cultures for making raw cultured vegetables, cultured butter, and sour cream, as well as kefir starter for making traditional milk kefir, young coconut kefir, and kefir cheese. Body Ecology also has fermented probiotic liquids (**InnergyBiotic, Coco Biotic, Whole Grains Biotic,** and **Dong Quai**). Dilute these liquids with sparkling mineral water and they make an ideal replacement for soft drinks when sweetened with Body Ecology's **Stevia Liquid Concentrate**.

Potent Proteins (100% fermented protein powder with 50% fermented spirulina) is a very sour, very potent way to nourish your liver, increase iron and magnesium levels, and significantly boost energy. It provides powerful probiotic benefits.

Raw cultured vegetables are now available in many stores around the country. There are also private "artisans" who make them and will ship to you.
  (See **www.bodyecology.com** for listings.)
Raw miso*
Raw natto (no MSG)*

FRUIT

Black currant juice from Austria (Austria's Finest
Naturally: **www.austriasfinestnaturally.com**)
Cranberries, fresh or frozen
Cranberry juice concentrate, pure and unsweetened
Lemons, fresh
Limes, fresh
Pomegranate juice or from concentrate
Noni, mangosteen, and acai juices, unsweetened (Genesis
Today: **www.genesistoday.com**)

GRAINS

(Remember to soak 8–24 hours)
Amaranth buckwheat (also called kasha)
Cream of Buckwheat cereal
(Pocono: **www.poconofoods.com**)
Millet
Puffed Millet Cereal, dry
(Arrowhead Mills: **www.arrowheadmills.com**)
Quinoa and Quinoa Flakes
(Ancient Harvest: **www.quinoa.net**)

STEVIA, SALT, HERBS, AND SPICES

Stevia: Body Ecology's own great-tasting liquid herbal
concentrate with no aftertaste.
Seasoning salts: Herbamare and Trocomare (A.Vogel: **www.
avogel.com**)
Garden herbs (fresh or dried). All traditional land herbs and
spices are on the B.E.D, including antifungal herbs like
cinnamon, coriander, curry, garlic, ginger, and turmeric.
Seasonings from the ocean (Maine Coast Sea Seasonings:
www.seaveg.com): Dulse, Dulse with Garlic, Kelp
with Cayenne (good substitute for salt and pepper).
Sea salt: The special sea salts we use in our Body Ecology
test kitchens are the most medicinal of salts and have
a superior "vibrational energy." We recommend you
use fine-grind and gray Celtic sea salt for cooking and

Hawaiian Deep Sea Salt at the table (Selina Naturally: **www.SelinaNaturally.com**).

━━∿∿∿━━

LAND VEGETABLES

All land vegetables except for cooked beets, mung bean sprouts, mushrooms (dried shiitake is okay), parsnips, green peppers, yams, and potatoes (red skin is okay)

━━∿∿∿━━

NUTS AND SEEDS

Always soaked and dehydrated

━━∿∿∿━━

OCEAN VEGETABLES

Agar, arame, dulse, hijiki, kelp, kombu, nori, sea palm, and wakame (Maine Coast Sea Vegetables: **www.seaveg. com**; Eden: **www.edenfoods.com**; and other brands)

━━∿∿∿━━

ORGANIC, UNREFINED OILS

Extra-virgin olive oil (Rallis [**www.rallisoliveoil.com**] has a premium, early-harvest *extra*-extra-virgin oil with a nearly flawless <0.14% acidity—needless to say, it is delicious and our absolute favorite)

Wild Alaskan Sockeye Salmon Oil (Vital Choice: **www.vitalchoice.com**)

Coconut oil

Pumpkin seed oil (Austria's Finest Naturally: **www. austriasfinestnaturally.com**)

X-Factor Gold High-Vitamin Butter Oil and Blue Ice Fermented Cod Liver Oil (both from Green Pasture: **www.greenpasture.org**)

Fish oil

Flax seed oil (Barlean's Organic Oils: **www.barleans.com**)

Flax with borage

The Essential Woman or Omega Man (both from Barlean's Organic Oils: **www.barleans.com**)

Macadamia nut oil

Red palm oil

━━∿∿∿━━

SALAD DRESSINGS AND CONDIMENTS

Mustards made with apple cider vinegar (Tree of Life's Whole Grain, Eden's mustard, Anne's Original Mountain Herb, Zake's Fire Country, True Natural Taste organic mustards: 800-559-2998)

Cindy's Kitchen Organic Creamy Miso salad dressing (**www.cindyskitchen.com**)

Spectrum salad dressings (**www.spectrumorganics.com**)

―❧―

TEAS

(Read labels carefully. There are many excellent herbal teas available, but green tea is an excellent choice. Avoid teas with citric acid and from fruits like raspberry; raspberry leaf, stem, or root is fine.)

Body Ecology's **Tea Concentrates**

Traditional Medicinals Weightless, Organic Ginger Aid, Organic Mother's Milk, Organic Echinacea Plus, Organic Echinacea Elder, Pau d'Arco, Organic Chamomile, Organic Raspberry Leaf (**www.traditionalmedicinals.com**)

―❧―

PERSONAL-CARE PRODUCTS

(Antimicrobial)

Thursday Plantation Tea Tree Suppositories (**www.thursdayplantation.com**)

Tea tree oil castile soap, dental floss, shampoo, mouthwash, and lip balm

NutriBiotic Dental Gel (**www.nutribiotic.com**)

Desert Essence Natural Tea Tree Oil & Neem Toothpaste (**www.desertessence.com**)

ProSeed Feminine Rinse (douche concentrate); ProSeed Nail Rescue (antifungal nail formula); ProSeed Healthy Gums (all from Imhotep, Inc.: **www.imhotepinc.com**)

Vita-Myr Zinc-Plus Toothpaste (herbal toothpaste with myrrh, clove, and grapefruit seed extract) (**www. vitamyr.com**)

―❧―

ANTIFUNGAL, ANTIVIRAL, ANTIBACTERIAL IMMUNE BOOSTERS

Oil of oregano
ProSeed Soothing Ear Drops
(Imhotep, Inc.: **www.imhotepinc.com**)
Olive leaf extract

—~~—

OTHER VALUABLE PRODUCTS

Body Ecology's **Vitality SuperGreen™** (preferred to a multiple vitamin, it is designed to help restore your inner ecosystem and supply a wide spectrum of easily digested nutrients)

Body Ecology's **Ocean Plant Extract™** (nourishes the thyroid to increase energy for healing, helps eliminate mercury, and protects against radiation— a must for pregnant women and those with an underactive thyroid)

Body Ecology's **LivAmend™** (helps support a healthy liver, increases bile flow, and improves bowel elimination)

Body Ecology's **Ancient Earth Minerals™** (chelated from ancient plant matter; and an excellent source of energy minerals, trace elements, and amino acids)

Body Ecology's **EcoBloom™** (100% natural chicory extract, a prebiotic to feed friendly flora; can be added to salad dressings, drinks, baked goods, and cultured foods before fermenting)

Genesis Today's 4 Fiber (has flax seeds, hemp seeds, noni fiber, and excellent herbs to promote better elimination; **www.genesistoday.com**)

Lecithin granules (tossed into a salad or salad dressing, this adds creaminess, aids fat metabolism, and is good for the brain and nervous system)

Morningstar Minerals Energy Boost 70 (a liquid fulvic acid, chelated from ancient plant matter, it's a great tasteless liquid source of minerals, trace elements, and amino acids that nourish your adrenals and thyroid . . . add to any food or drink you prepare; **www. msminerals.com**)

Morningstar Minerals Vitality Boost HA (great to implant after your colon cleansing sessions; **www.msminerals. com**)

Xanthan gum (add to salad for thickening; see page 299)

KEFIR PRODUCTS

(Commercially produced are of poor quality and cannot compare to fresh, delicious homemade kefir)

Body Ecology's **Kefir Starter** (for homemade milk kefir or for fermenting the liquid and spoon-meat of the young coconut)

PROBIOTICS

Your local health-food store carries many excellent probiotic supplements. They all are far more effective when taken with the fermented foods on the Body Ecology Diet. Our favorites include Natren's Life Start (*Bifidus infantis;* **www.natren.com**) and New Chapter Probiotic Anti-Aging, Probiotic Colon, Probiotic Immunity, Probiotic Cleanse, and Probiotic All-Flora (**www.newchapter.com**).

OTHER BOOKS YOU'LL WANT TO READ

The Baby Boomer Diet: Body Ecology's Guide to Growing Younger, by Donna Gates with Lyndi Schrecengost

The Stevia Cookbook: Cooking with Nature's Calorie-Free Sweetener, by Ray Sahelian, M.D., and Donna Gates

*These foods are not tolerated by everyone. Avoid them the first six weeks, then introduce them by rotating them into your diet once every four days and eat them with alkaline, non-starchy vegetables; avoid eating them alone.

Many of the products listed here are available in your local health-food store. Body Ecology's products (appearing in bold) are available online at **www.bodyecology.com** or by calling 866-4BE-DIET (423-3438). Your local health-food store can also order them for you.

Appendix B

Bibliography

Part I: Introduction: A Silent Spring Within

Chapters 1, 2, 3, and 4

Annechild, Annette, and Laura Johnson. *Yeast-Free Living*. New York, NY, The Putnam Publishing Group, 1986.

Carson, Rachel. *Silent Spring*. Boston, MA, Houghton Mifflin Company, 1987.

Chaitow, Leon, D.O., M.D. *Candida Albicans: Could Yeast Be Your Problem?* Rochester, VT, Healing Arts Press, 1988.

Crook, William G., M.D. *The Yeast Connection: A Medical Breakthrough*. Jackson, TN, Professional Books, 1985.

De Schepper, Luc, M.D., Ph.D., C.A. *Candida*. Santa Monica, CA, 1986. (213-828-4480)

Finnegan, John. *Yeast Disorders: An Understanding and Nutritional Therapy*. Mill Valley, CA, Elysian Arts, 1989.

Glasser, Ronald J. *The Body Is The Hero*. New York, NY, Bantam Books, 1979.

Lappe, Marc. *When Antibiotics FAIL: Restoring the Ecology of the Body*. Berkeley, CA, North Atlantic Books, 1986.

Lorenzani, Shirley S., Ph.D. *Candida: A Twentieth Century Disease*. New Canaan, CT, Keats Publishing, Inc., 1986.

Miller, Jonathon D., M.A., M.Div. *Candida Yeast: The Battle in Your Body*. Akron, OH, Lifecircle Publications, 1986.

Remington, Dennis W., M.D., and Barbara W. Higa, R.D. *Back to Health: A Comprehensive Medical and Nutritional Yeast Control Program.* Provo, UT, Vitality House International, Inc., 1987.

Robbins, John. *Diet for a New America.* Walpole, NH, Stillpoint Publishing, 1987. (800-847-4014)

Rochlitz, Steven. *Allergies And Candida: With The Physicist's Rapid Solution.* Setauket, NY, Human Ecology Balancing Sciences, Inc., 1989.

Schmidt, Michael A., Lendon H. Smith, and Keith W. Sehnert. *Beyond Antibiotics: Healthier Options for Families.* Berkeley, CA, North Atlantic Books, 1993.

Sehnert, Keith W., M.D. *The Garden Within: Acidophilus-Candida Connection.* Burlingame, CA, Health World, Inc., 1989.

Tenney, Louise. *Candida Albicans: A Nutritional Approach.* Provo, UT, Woodland Books, 1986.

Trowbridge, John P., M.D., and Morton Walker, D.P.M. *The Yeast Syndrome.* New York, NY, Bantam Books, 1986.

Part II: Principles of the Body Ecology Diet

Chapter 5 - The Principle of Expansion and Contraction

Aihara, Herman. *Basic Macrobiotics.* New York, NY, Japan Publications, Inc., 1985.

Garvy, John W., Jr., N.D., D.Ac. *Yin and Yang: Two Hands Clapping.* Newtonville, MA, Wellbeing Books, 1985.

Heidenry, Carolyn. *Making the Transition to a Macrobiotic Diet: A Beginner's Guide to the Natural Way of Health.* Wayne, NJ, Avery Publishing Group Inc., 1987.

Kushi, Michio, with Alex Jack. *The Book of Macrobiotics: The Universal Way of Health, Happiness, and Peace.* New York, NY, Japan Publications, Inc., 1989.

Kushi, Michio, edited by Marc Van Cauwenberghe, M.D. *Macrobiotic Home Remedies.* New York, NY, Japan Publications, Inc., 1985.

Lu, Henry C. *Chinese System of Food Cures: Prevention and Remedies.* New York, NY, Sterling Publishing Co., 1986.

Rogers, Sherry A., M.D. *You Are What You Ate: A Macrobiotic Way: An Rx for the Resistant Diseases of the 21st Century.* Syracuse, NY, Prestige Publishers, 1988.

Tara, William. *Macrobiotics and Human Behavior.* New York, NY, Japan Publications, Inc., 1984.

Chapter 6 - The Principle of Acid and Alkaline

Aihara, Herman. *Acid and Alkaline*. Oroville, CA, George Ohsawa Macrobiotic Foundation, 1986.

Chapter 9 - The Principle of Food Combining

Diamond, Harvey, and Marilyn Diamond. *Fit for Life*. New York, NY, Warner Books, 1985.

Diamond, Harvey, and Marilyn Diamond. *Fit for Life II: Living Health*. New York, NY, Warner Books, 1987.

Diamond, Marilyn. *A New Way of Eating*. New York, NY, Warner Books, 1987.

DuBelle, Lee. *Proper Food Combining Cookbook*. Phoenix, AZ, Lee DuBelle, P.O. Box 35860, 1984.

DuBelle, Lee. *Proper Food Combining Works: Living Testimony*. Phoenix, AZ, Lee DuBelle, P.O. Box 35860, 1986.

Fogel, Elaine. *The Food Combining Handbook and Cookbook*. Ontario, Canada, Mystery Laine Publishing, 1983.

Grant, Doris, and Jean Joice. *Food Combining for Health: A New Look at the Hay System*. Rochester, VT, Thorsons Publishing Group, 1984.

Grant, Doris, and Jean Joice. *Food Combining for Health: Get Fit with Foods That Don't Fight*. Rochester, VT, Thorsons Publishing Group, 1984.

Kahn, Pam, with Dennis Nelson. *Food Combining Recipe Book*. Santa Cruz, CA, The Plan, P.O. Box 872, 1986.

Mannix, Jeffrey. *Food Combining: The High-Energy Weight Loss Plan*. New York, NY, Contemporary Books, Inc., 1983.

Nelson, Dennis. *Food Combining Simplified: How to Get the Most from Your Food*. Santa Cruz, CA, The Plan, D. Nelson, P.O. Box 2302, 1985.

Null, Gary, and Staff. *Food Combining Handbook*. New York, NY, Jove Publications, Inc., 1973.

Shelton, Herbert M. *Food Combining Made Easy*. San Antonio, TX, Willow Publishing, Inc., 1982.

Smith, Esther L. *Good Foods That Go Together: The Official Cookbook of the Hay System*. New Canaan, CT, Keats Publishing, Inc., 1975.

Part III: Description of the Body Ecology Diet

Chapter 12 - What *Is* the Body Ecology Diet?

Finnegan, John. *The Facts About Fats: A Consumer's Guide to Good Oil*. Berkeley, CA, Celestial Arts Publishing, 1993.

Howard, Dr. Edward. *Enzyme Nutrition: The Food Enzyme Concept*. Wayne, NJ, Avery Publishing Group, Inc., 1985.

Jennings-Sauer, Cheryl. "The Egg's Return," *American Health*, April, 1988.

Roberts, H.J. *Aspartame (NutraSweet®) Is It Safe?* Philadelphia, PA, The Charles Press, Publishers, Inc., 1990.

Santillo, Humbart. *Food Enzymes: The Missing Link to Radiant Health*. Prescott Valley, AZ, Hohm Press, 1987.

Part IV: Rebuilding the Immune System

Chapter 18 - How to Care for Your Colon

Chaitow, Leon, N.D., D.O., and Natasha Trenev. *Probiotics: The Revolutionary, 'Friendly Bacteria' Way to Vital Health and Well-Being*. Hammersmith, London, Thorsons, 1990.

Gray, Robert. *The Colon Health Handbook: New Health Through Colon Rejuvenation*. Reno, NV, Emerald Publishing, 1986.

De Schepper, Luc, M.D., Ph.D., C.A. *Peak Immunity*. Santa Monica, CA, 1989. (213-828-4480)

Weinberger, Stanley. *Healing Within: The Complete Colon Health Guide*. Larkspur, CA, Colon Health Center, 1988.

Chapter 20 - How to Strengthen Your Immunity

Muramoto, Noboru B. *Natural Immunity: Insights on Diet and AIDS*. Oroville, CA, George Ohsawa Macrobiotic Foundation, 1988.

Tenney, Louise. *AIDS: A Nutritional Approach*. Provo, UT, Woodland Books, 1986.

Part V: Blood Type

Chapter 25 - The B.E.D. View of the Blood Type Theory

D'Adamo, Dr. James. *The D'Adamo Diet*. Toronto, Canada, McGraw-Hill Ryerson, 1989.

D'Adamo, Dr. James, with Allan Richards. *One Man's Food . . . Is Someone Else's Poison*. Toronto, Canada, Health Thru Herbs, Inc., 1980.

D'Adamo, Dr. Peter. *Eat Right for Your Type*. New York, NY, G.P. Putnam's Sons, 1996.

Nomi, Toshitaka, and Alexander Besher. *You Are Your Blood Type: The Biochemical Key to Unlocking the Secrets of Your Personality*. New York, NY, Pocket Books, 1988.

Index

The Body Ecology Mission

As the leader in fermented foods and nutrition, our mission at BODY ECOLOGY is to change the way the world eats, thus ending disease. We want every home in America to be using the healthy foods we recommend in this book. We want all children to be born with perfect health. With advances in modern genomics coupled with Body Ecology's Seven Universal Principles and our BED foods . . . especially fermented foods . . . this can be our future.

Please help us spread the word:

✔ Eating a variety of cultured foods found all around the world helps create a healthy inner ecosystem and contributes to a long, healthy lifespan.

✔ Organic, unrefined seed oils, coconut oil, extra-virgin olive oil, raw butter, and raw cream are the best fats to eat. Avoid bleached, refined, and deodorized vegetable oils commonly found in most foods. Also avoid margarine.

✔ Stevia is an excellent choice to satisfy your sweet tooth.

✔ Taking an alkaline, mineral-rich superfoods formula is even better than man-made supplements for reversing protein, mineral, and essential fatty acid deficiencies.

✔ Raw apple cider vinegar is the only really healthy vinegar.

✔ Ocean vegetables and organic land vegetables should make up a significant portion of each meal.

✔ Cold-water fish, free-range poultry, and eggs from free-running, fertile chickens are your best sources of animal protein.

BEDROK and Autism

Body Ecology Diet Recovering Our Kids

The Body Ecology Diet (BED), developed by Donna Gates, has been in use for over 15 years to address immune-system issues, including viral and fungal infections, various autoimmune diseases, nutritional deficiencies, and digestive disorders (IBS, ulcerative colitis, and Crohn's disease). For the past several years it has been used experimentally within the autism community with very positive results. BEDROK children improve dramatically when their parents introduce our principles and our foods into their way of life.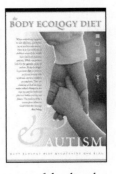

The BED views autism as a combination of disorders—all correctable. A gut-brain infection in the early stages of the disorder distances the child from his surroundings. The goal of dietary intervention is to bring him back into our world and back to his true self.

Donna Gates has a passion for helping children. BEDROK (Body Ecology Diet Recovering Our Kids) is a program she is developing together with parents of children with autism. BEDROK has a strong spiritual component to it. Donna truly believes that the children coming into our world today are highly evolved beings and need to be treated as such. She explains, "Our planet is in such turmoil at the moment, and many children in this new generation carry priceless information and solutions to our most serious problems. But these highly evolved souls will come of age unable to fulfill their missions on earth unless we correct the conditions that threaten to hold them back."

Autism has multiple causes, including:

- Undetected infections (fungal and viral)
- Environmental toxins inherited from several previous generations
- Weak endocrine organs (adrenal and thyroid)
- Blocked detoxification pathways that prevent toxins from leaving the body
- Congested livers
- Nutritional deficiencies coupled with vulnerable immune systems due to the lack of an "inner ecosystem"

All these form a complex disorder that takes our children away from us and ultimately will prevent them from accomplishing their spiritual purpose. It is our responsibility to bring them back. The world needs this generation; we can't afford to lose them.

Please visit us at www.bodyecology.com to learn more about Body Ecology Diet research on autism, chat about autism and ADD, and browse a wide range of information and products to recover your inner ecology. Or call 866-4BE-DIET.

Acknowledgments

Since 1994 when the first edition of *The Body Ecology Diet* was published, many wonderful people have contributed to making it a bestseller. To my friends, family, Certified Body Ecologists, and business associates, I offer my heartfelt thanks. And to those of you I haven't met, I am grateful beyond words for your help in carrying this work forward by sharing my book with others.

I will always appreciate the help of Linda Schatz and Heidi Wohl, who came into my life at an extraordinarily busy time. I was struggling with how to get all the information that was stored in my mind written down in an organized manner to help the growing number of people who had heard about my work. Both women had come to my classes to learn how to heal themselves of candidiasis. While they say they are grateful for what I gave them, it is I, and you the readers, who are benefiting enormously from their selfless, consistent determination in helping bring this book to fruition.

There are two special men I absolutely must thank, Richard Thomas and his son Jim, who made a long-held wish come true. My secret wish was for a restaurant where people could experience a Body Ecology meal, lovingly prepared and served, featuring coconut and organic, unrefined oils, organic grains and vegetables, free-range chicken, and even ocean and cultured vegetables. Today, such a restaurant exists. In addition to serving delicious meals at the R. Thomas Deluxe Grill on Peachtree Street in Atlanta, the restaurant delivers Body Ecology meals and cultured vegetables to local health-food stores, making it easy for BEDers to stay on The Diet.

Finally, to the One Who created us all, Who has patiently watched us make mistakes yet has never given up on us . . . and Who is (with strict love) guiding us back into the Light, I owe my deepest and most sincere gratitude.

This book is dedicated to those who have the discernment to recognize the truth and the courage to live it.

Donna Gates

ABOUT THE AUTHORS

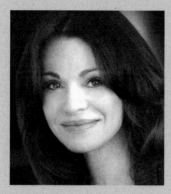

Donna Gates has helped hundreds of thousands of people overcome immune-system disorders and other health issues and achieve peak health. She is known as the teacher to the teachers, and her insights continue to guide many of today's most renowned natural-health physicians and other professionals. An expert on candidiasis (CRC) and related immune disorders, she has done extensive research on how these debilitating conditions affect the body, mind, and spirit. She developed and tested the Body Ecology Diet on many different people, who have all improved their health by following the basic principles of The Diet.

Donna is a nutritional consultant, home economist, and founder of Body Ecology, Inc., a leading nutrition company. She has studied with the top macrobiotic teachers and graduated from Lima Osawa's cooking academy in Japan. She holds an M.Ed. in Counseling from Loyola University and a B.S. in Early Childhood Development from the University of Georgia. Donna is credited with leading some of the most important innovations in natural health, including inventing young coconut kefir, being at the forefront of probiotics and fermented foods, and bringing stevia/reb A (powder and liquid), along with other products, into the US.

Donna's free newsletter, available at www.BodyEcology.com, is one of the most widely read and respected natural-health publications in the world. Her eagerly anticipated book *The Baby Boomer Diet* is expected to revolutionize the way we think about aging.

Linda Schatz is a professional writer and editor. She is the coauthor of *Managing by Influence* (Prentice Hall) and has been a newswriter for ABC News and Good Morning America. She also coaches authors on how to write books and book proposals. Her specialties are self-help titles in areas such as health, nutrition, and business. Linda holds an M.A. in Communication from Stanford University and a B.S. in Journalism from the University of California, Berkeley.

www.bodyecology.com

Stay Connected with Body Ecology!

You can make a difference in the world by simply joining Body Ecology in its mission to change the way the world eats. The Body Ecology tribe can be found on Facebook and Twitter.

www.facebook.com/bodyecology

BodyEcology

The Body Ecology Facebook fan page is teeming with activity. Great health topics are addressed, and support with helpful suggestions are offered from thousands of health-minded "friends and fans." How can you impact your family, friends, and community? Start living the Body Ecology lifestyle! Learn our system of health and healing, and put it into practice step by step – just watch the difference it will make in your life and in the lives of those around your. Learn more on Facebook and Twitter!

Subscribe to Body Ecology's FREE e-Newsletter

The Body Ecology Health & Wellness e-Newsletter is cherished by readers around the world and widely considered one of THE most important newsletters available. It's an essential read for anyone committed to improving their health. Once you subscribe, you will find health insights and solutions with a strong focus on natural and alternative health angles – 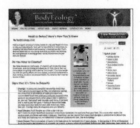 long before you read them elsewhere. In fact, many of the world's most renowned and respected natural health physicians and dietary experts have referred to Body Ecology to learn essential insights that are then incorporated into their own health programs and publications.

Even more important, the health and wellness insights you'll discover in every free issue REALLY WORK. The natural/dietary-health-focused articles you'll read are a combination of scientific research, common sense, and factual data. Tens of thousands of people have genuinely seen their health *dramatically improve* through the well-researched and easy-to-understand insights provided by Body Ecology.

Sign up today for FREE at www.BodyEcology.com

We hope you enjoyed this Hay House book.
If you would like to receive a free catalogue featuring additional
Hay House books and products, or if you would like information
about the Hay Foundation, please contact:

Hay House UK Ltd
292B Kensal Road • London W10 5BE
Tel: (44) 20 8962 1230; Fax: (44) 20 8962 1239
www.hayhouse.co.uk

***

Published and distributed in the United States of America by:
Hay House, Inc. • PO Box 5100 • Carlsbad, CA 92018-5100
Tel: (1) 760 431 7695 or (1) 800 654 5126;
Fax: (1) 760 431 6948 or (1) 800 650 5115
www.hayhouse.com

***

Published and distributed in Australia by:
Hay House Australia Ltd • 18/36 Ralph Street • Alexandria, NSW 2015
Tel: (61) 2 9669 4299, Fax: (61) 2 9669 4144
www.hayhouse.com.au

***

Published and distributed in the Republic of South Africa by:
Hay House SA (Pty) Ltd • PO Box 990 • Witkoppen 2068
Tel/Fax: (27) 11 467 8904
www.hayhouse.co.za

***

Published and distributed in India by:
Hay House Publishers India • Muskaan Complex • Plot No.3
B-2 • Vasant Kunj • New Delhi - 110 070
Tel: (91) 11 41761620; Fax: (91) 11 41761630
www.hayhouse.co.in

***

Distributed in Canada by:
Raincoast • 9050 Shaughnessy St • Vancouver, BC V6P 6E5
Tel: (1) 604 323 7100
Fax: (1) 604 323 2600

***

Sign up via the Hay House UK website to receive the Hay House
online newsletter and stay informed about what's going on with your
favourite authors. You'll receive bimonthly announcements
about discounts and offers, special events, product highlights,
free excerpts, giveaways, and more!
www.hayhouse.co.uk

JOIN THE HAY HOUSE FAMILY

As the leading self-help, mind, body and spirit publisher in the UK, we'd like to welcome you to our family so that you can enjoy all the benefits our website has to offer.

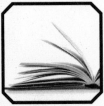 **EXTRACTS** from a selection of your favourite author titles

 **COMPETITIONS, PRIZES & SPECIAL OFFERS** Win extracts, money off, downloads and so much more

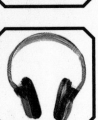 **LISTEN** to a range of radio interviews and our latest audio publications

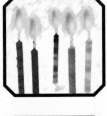 **CELEBRATE YOUR BIRTHDAY** An inspiring gift will be sent your way

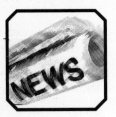 **LATEST NEWS** Keep up with the latest news from and about our authors

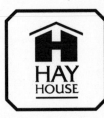 **ATTEND OUR AUTHOR EVENTS** Be the first to hear about our author events

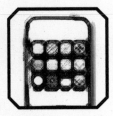 **iPHONE APPS** Download your favourite app for your iPhone

 HAY HOUSE INFORMATION Ask us anything, all enquiries answered

join us online at **www.hayhouse.co.uk**

 292B Kensal Road, London W10 5BE
T: 020 8962 1230 E: info@hayhouse.co.uk